Necropsy Guide for Dogs, Cats,
and Small Mammals

This book is dedicated to John M. King, who wrote The Necropsy Book, and taught us all about the art of the necropsy.

Necropsy Guide for Dogs, Cats, and Small Mammals

Edited by

Sean P. McDonough
DVM, PhD, Diplomate ACVP
Cornell University
Ithaca, NY

Teresa Southard
DVM, PhD, Diplomate ACVP
Cornell University
Ithaca, NY

WILEY Blackwell

This edition first published 2017 © 2017 John Wiley & Sons, Inc

Editorial Offices
1606 Golden Aspen Drive, Suites 103 and 104, Ames, Iowa 50010, USA
The Atrium, Southern Gate, Chichester, West Sussex, PO19 8SQ, UK
1606 Golden Aspen Drive, Suites 103 and 104, Ames, Iowa 50010, USA

For details of our global editorial offices, for customer services and for information about how to apply for permission to reuse the copyright material in this book please see our website at www.wiley.com/wiley-blackwell.

Library of Congress Cataloging-in-Publication Data

Names: McDonough, Sean P., editor. | Southard, Teresa, editor.
Title: Necropsy guide for dogs, cats, and small mammals / edited by Sean P. McDonough, Teresa Southard.
Description: Ames, Iowa, USA : John Wiley & Sons Inc., 2017. | Includes bibliographical references and index.
Identifiers: LCCN 2016036895 | ISBN 9781119115656 (pbk.) | ISBN 9781119115670 (ePub) | ISBN 9781119115663 (Adobe PDF)
Subjects: LCSH: Veterinary autopsy. | Dogs–Autopsy. | Cats–Autopsy. | MESH: Autopsy–veterinary | Autopsy–methods |
    Dissection–veterinary | Dogs | Cats
Classification: LCC SF769 .N43 2017 | NLM SF 769 | DDC 636.089/60759–dc23
LC record available at https://lccn.loc.gov/2016036895

A catalogue record for this book is available from the British Library.

Wiley also publishes its books in a variety of electronic formats. Some content that appears in print may not be available in electronic books.

Set in 10/12pt Warnock by SPi Global, Pondicherry, India

10 9 8 7 6 5 4 3 2 1

Brief Contents

Contents

List of Contributors

Elizabeth L. Buckles, DVM, PhD, Diplomate ACVP
Department of Biomedical Sciences
College of Veterinary Medicine
Cornell University

Gerald E. Duhamel, DVM, PhD, Diplomate ACVP
Department of Biomedical Sciences,
College of Veterinary Medicine,
Cornell University

Kathleen M. Kelly, DVM, PhD, Diplomate ACVP
Department of Biomedical Sciences
College of Veterinary Medicine
Cornell University

Andrew D. Miller, DVM, Diplomate ACVP
Department of Biomedical Sciences
College of Veterinary Medicine
Cornell University

Jeanine Peters-Kennedy, DVM, Diplomate ACVP, Diplomate ACVD
Department of Biomedical Sciences
College of Veterinary Medicine
Cornell University

Foreword

"Internists know everything and do nothing; Surgeons know nothing and do everything; Pathologists know everything and do everything, but it's too late."

This saying is popular among veterinary and medical students and reflects some common stereotypes about the different disciplines in our professions. We will let the internists and surgeons speak for themselves, but as pathologists, we like to think that our knowledge base is equivalent to an internist and our technical skills rival those of a surgeon. And we concede that our efforts are not going to help the patient on the necropsy table; however, the work of the pathologist is not too late to make a big impact. A necropsy examination is a simple, cost-effective, broad spectrum diagnostic procedure that requires no advanced training or high priced equipment and can provide information beneficial to the animal's family and veterinary team, as well our overall understanding of disease processes (animal and human), which could potentially save other lives.

Despite the benefits of a necropsy, this procedure is rarely performed, and often not even considered. Here at Cornell, only a small percentage of the animals that die or are euthanized in the small animal hospital are submitted for necropsy. In human medicine, the autopsy rate has drastically declined over the past few decades. Before the 1970s, 30–40% of all human hospital deaths were investigated by autopsy but by 2005, the rate had fallen to less than 10%, with almost no autopsies performed at hospitals that are not affiliated with an academic institution.

Necropsies are not performed for a variety of reasons. The death of a companion animal is always an emotional time and broaching the subject of a necropsy may seem insensitive. However, input from the clinicians at the Cornell University Hospital for Animals suggests that if owners believe something positive can come from the death of their pet, especially knowledge that could potentially help other animals, they are much more likely to consent to a postmortem examination. Also, many veterinarians, especially at tertiary care facilities, share the belief of physicians that the advent of newer diagnostic techniques and powerful imaging modalities makes the necropsy or autopsy obsolete. However, despite the advances in medical technology, the rate of diagnostic errors remains high. Up to 10% of autopsies reveal a misdiagnosis that would likely have affected patient outcome and the cause of death is misdiagnosed in almost 25% of cases. Our personal experience with necropsies reveals similar percentages of misdiagnoses in veterinary medicine.

The goal of this book is to provide veterinary students and small animal practitioners, as well as pathology residents and pathologists, a guide for performing a necropsy, including a step-by-step tutorial of the basic necropsy procedure, a review of the anatomy and dissection techniques for each organ system, and information on collecting tissues for additional testing. We hope more veterinarians will take advantage of the unique continuing educational opportunity the necropsy affords them.

Acknowledgments

We are grateful to everyone who helped make this book a reality, particularly Jodie Gerdin, who got this whole project started; Karyn Bischoff, James Morrisey, Ashleigh Newman, Pamela Schenck, Belinda Thompson, and Jimmy Tran, who contributed their knowledge, time and resources; and the Cornell pathology residents and necropsy students who were patient with us as we interrupted their work to take pictures. Photograph contributors for this book include: Don Schlafer, Ana Alcaraz, Roger Panciera, Gavin Hitchener, May Tse, Nick Vitale, Jimmy Tran, Stacy Rine, Alex Molesan, and Heather Daverio.

About the Companion Website

This book is accompanied by a companion website:

www.wilcy.com/go/mcdonough/necropsy

The website includes:

- Video of necropsy being performed.

Part I

Necropsy Fundamentals

1

Introduction to the Necropsy

1.1   What is a Necropsy?

A necropsy is a postmortem examination. By convention, this term is typically used to denote a postmortem examination of a non-human animal, and the term "autopsy" is used for a postmortem examination of a human; however, the terms are essentially interchangeable, and some veterinary pathologists have argued for the use of a common term to increase communication in the age of "one medicine." Both terms are derived from Greek words: autopsy is from the word *autopsia*, meaning the act of seeing for one's self; necropsy is from the words *nekros* meaning dead and the suffix *-opsis* meaning sight. The word autopsy was used in the 1600s, and the word necropsy did not appear until about 200 years later, most likely to replace the two-word term *autopsia cadavaria*, or to look for oneself at a dead body. We chose the term *necropsy* for this book because it is the term we use at Cornell, where the word is deeply rooted in the long-standing tradition of veterinary pathology.

The term necropsy can be used broadly to encompass the entire set of diagnostic procedures that occur after an animal dies; however, in this book we will use the term to denote the macroscopic or gross examination of the carcass and the process of collecting tissues for histopathology and other ancillary tests. At Cornell and most diagnostic laboratories, the fee for a necropsy includes both gross examination and microscopic evaluation of the tissues collected during the necropsy; however, for a reduced fee, the formalin fixed tissues collected by a referring veterinarian or scientist can be processed and examined histologically (we call this type of case a "necropsy in a bottle"). If the clinician is willing to do the necropsy and collect the tissues, the necropsy in a bottle option is often an economically attractive alternative to shipping the carcass to a diagnostic lab.

In this text, the term *prosector* will be used for the person performing the necropsy.

1.2   Why do a Necropsy?

Necropsies are performed to determine or confirm the cause of death or reason for a condition necessitating euthanasia. A necropsy may be requested by an owner, a veterinarian, a drug or vaccine company, a biomedical researcher, or a law enforcement or other government agency. The common reasons for necropsy requests at Cornell are shown in Table 1.1.

1.3   What Information Can and Cannot Be Gained from a Necropsy

A necropsy can result in a definitive diagnosis, a presumptive diagnosis or, if there are no gross lesions, will at least rule out some possible diagnoses.

Necropsy Guide for Dogs, Cats, and Small Mammals, First Edition. Edited by Sean P. McDonough and Teresa Southard.
© 2017 John Wiley & Sons, Inc. Published 2017 by John Wiley & Sons, Inc.
Companion Website: www.wiley.com/go/mcdonough/necropsy

Table 1.1 Reasons necropsies are requested.

Owner	Gain peace of mind, especially about a decision to euthanize
	Rule in or out infectious/toxic cause when other animals are at risk
	Suspicion of malicious action by another party (usually the neighbor)
	Suspicion of veterinary malpractice
	Concern about zoonotic disease (rabies)
	Insurance reasons (most common in horses)
Veterinarian	Find answers in a confusing or atypical case
	Confirm a suspected diagnosis
	Examine surgical sites or retrieve implanted devices
	Collect data about a condition of interest
Drug or Vaccine Company	Determine if drug or vaccine caused illness or death
Biomedical Researcher	Investigate cause of unexpected death in animal on a study
	Compare control and experimental animals at end of study
Law Enforcement or Government Agency	Animal harmed or killed during police activity
	Suspicion of criminal cruelty or neglect
	Suspicion of a pet-food related toxicity

Necropsies are particularly rewarding when they reveal pathognomonic gross lesions. These gross changes are specific for a particular disease entity and can often allow the prosector to make a definitive diagnosis with no need for additional testing. Some of these conditions are illustrated in Figures 1.1–1.6. Unfortunately, these cases make up only about 10% of our caseload at Cornell.

In another small portion of cases, again roughly 10%, the necropsy reveals no lesions to suggest a cause of death, either because all organs are grossly normal or because the body is decomposed to the point that lesions cannot be distinguished from the processes of decay. Abortions and neonatal deaths are our lowest yield necropsies, and often these cases go unresolved even with complete ancillary testing. Causes of death that typically have minimal or no gross lesions include metabolic derangements, many toxicities (especially neurotoxins), and cardiac arrhythmias.

For the vast majority of cases, the necropsy provides some clues as to the disease process, allows for a presumptive diagnosis, and directs sampling for additional tests that, in many cases, will yield a definitive diagnosis.

1.4 When to Refer a Necropsy

Anyone who has a good grasp of normal veterinary anatomy can perform a necropsy (especially if they read this book!) No advanced training is required; however, before beginning, a practitioner should make a realistic assessment of their ability to perform a particular necropsy. There are certain types of necropsies that are best handled by specialists in facilities specifically designed for postmortem examinations. Necropsies should be referred to a diagnostic laboratory with board certified pathologists in the following circumstances:

1) Cases where a client expresses concerns about your veterinary care of the patient
2) Cases which are part of a legal dispute (forensic necropsy)
3) Cases with strong suspicion of a zoonotic agent, such as rabies or tularemia
4) Cases involving unfamiliar species, such as non-human primates, reptiles, and birds.

Veterinarians sometimes open up the body to look for obvious gross lesions and, if none are detected, pack up the opened carcass and send it to us for a "second look necropsy."

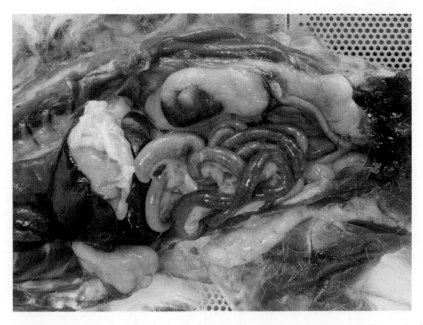

Figure 1.1 Segmental hemorrhagic enteritis in this 8 week old kitten is virtually diagnostic for panleukopenia caused by feline parvovirus. The lesion in puppies with canine parvovirus infection is similar.

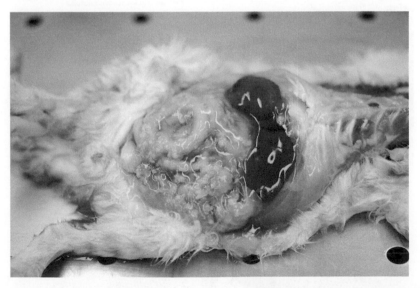

Figure 1.2 The wet form of feline infectious peritonitis often causes bright yellow, thick peritoneal effusion and multifocal tan to white plaques on the serosal surfaces.

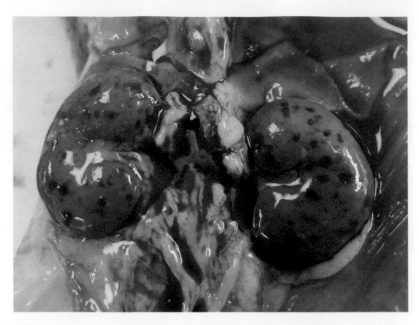

Figure 1.3 Dark red foci on the capsular surface of the kidneys in a newborn puppy usually indicates infection with canine herpesvirus.

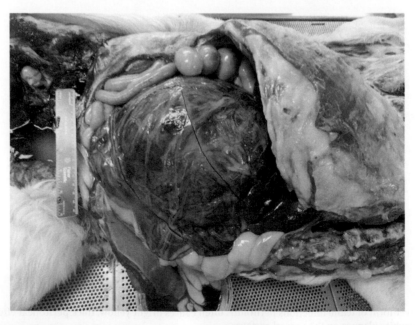

Figure 1.4 The gross finding of a distended, rotated, congested stomach is characteristic of gastric dilatation volvulus in a dog.

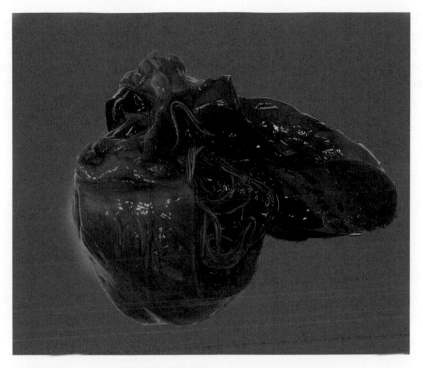

Figure 1.5 Long, slender tan nematode parasites in the right side of the heart and pulmonary artery are pathognomonic for heart worm infection (dirofilariasis).

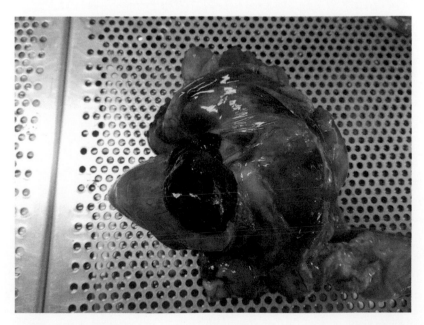

Figure 1.6 A dark red mass associated with the right atrium, with or without rupture and hemopericardium, in a dog strongly supports a diagnosis of hemangiosarcoma.

Opening the body cavities leads to significant artifactual changes in the color and consistency of the viscera and may interfere with both gross interpretation of lesions and the ability to collect optimal samples for additional testing. The preferred course of action at this point would be to continue with the necropsy, take digital photos, and send us the photos along with formalin-fixed (and fresh, if appropriate) samples.

2

Necropsy Basics

This chapter provides some background information for the prosector before starting the necropsy, including essential supplies, safety considerations, documentation of necropsy findings, and the physiology and gross manifestations of postmortem change.

2.1 Necropsy Facilities

The necropsy procedure does not require a specialized facility. Large animal veterinarians routinely perform necropsies in a pasture or a barn. In a small animal clinic or laboratory setting, a stainless steel work table with running water and plumbed to a sanitary sewer line is ideal. The area chosen should be easy to clean and disinfect. The necropsy should be performed at a time and place where there are minimal distractions and foot traffic so as to minimize the chances of cross contamination.

2.2 Necropsy Equipment

The instruments and supplies needed to perform a necropsy are relatively few and inexpensive. The major expense is the investment of an adequate amount of time to perform a complete necropsy. A kit assembled beforehand can facilitate the necropsy process. Next is a suggested list of equipment and supplies:

1) *Sharp blade for cutting soft tissue: Knife, scalpel*
A sharp blade is the most important tool for the prosector. The choice between a knife and a scalpel should depend on availability, size of the animal and personal preference. A good knife will hold its edge better than a scalpel blade and can be sharpened as needed. Correctly sharpening a knife requires considerable skill and patience. A flat ground blade made of stainless steel is a bit harder to sharpen but the cutting edge will usually hold up better than a double angle edge. A wooden handle is porous and may absorb pathogens, so a synthetic handle that can be easily disinfected is preferred. A steel is essential to hone the blade after sharpening and to revive the edge after cutting for a while. The steel should be at least as long as your knife blade. Hold the knife crossways against the steel and tilt the blade until the cutting edge meets the shaft of the steel at a 22.5° angle (hint: hold the blade perpendicular to the steel, then cut the angle in half to 45°; cut the angle in half again to reach the correct angle). Gently draw the blade towards you while gliding it down the length of the steel (Fig. 2.1). Repeat 10 to 12 times on each side and then rinse and wipe the blade with a cloth to remove any metal filings.

A scalpel is a good choice for the necropsy of a puppy, kitten, or small mammal. For a medium to large sized animal, a knife is usually the best choice for opening the carcass,

Necropsy Guide for Dogs, Cats, and Small Mammals, First Edition. Edited by Sean P. McDonough and Teresa Southard.
© 2017 John Wiley & Sons, Inc. Published 2017 by John Wiley & Sons, Inc.
Companion Website: www.wiley.com/go/mcdonough/necropsy

while a scalpel can be used for more delicate dissection of the organs.

2) *Sturdy instrument for cutting bone and removing the brain: Bone cutting forceps, hedge clippers, pruning shears, oscillating saw*

A complete necropsy requires cutting the bones of the ribs and skull to access the viscera, as well as the femur to examine the bone marrow. In kittens, puppies, and small mammals, bone forceps (Fig. 2.2) or strong scissors (e.g., poultry scissors) are sufficient for these tasks. Bone forceps are also the tool of choice for cutting the ribs of small dogs and most cats, and can be used to open the skulls of these animals as well. These tools are often referred to as rongeurs, but rongeurs have a curved tip for scooping out bone, while bone forceps have a sharp, cutting edge. Removal of the brain in most adult cats and dogs is most efficiently performed with an oscillating saw (Fig. 2.3). For medium to large sized dogs hedge clippers are the instrument of choice for cutting ribs. (Fig. 2.4) A hand saw can also be used to cut ribs and to open skulls of large dogs. An instrument called a T tool (Fig. 2.5) is very helpful in prying the skull cap off after the initial cuts through the bone have been made with an oscillating saw.

3) *Dissection instruments: Forceps, scissors*

Forceps and scissors are helpful tools for dissecting and collecting soft tissue. Rat tooth forceps cause less tissue artifact in histologic sections than forceps that crush the tissue. Scissors with at least one blunt tip are very useful in opening the intestine and other tubular organs without damaging the tissue. The size of the dissection instruments should be scaled to the size of the animal.

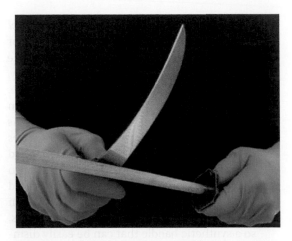

Figure 2.1 To hone the edge on a knife, place the edge of the knife against the sharpening steel at an angle of approximately 20 degree and pull the knife across the steel in a slight arc. Repeat this motion 10 times, alternating sides of the blade.

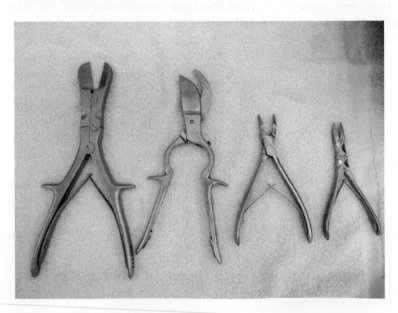

Figure 2.2 In cats and small dogs, bone cutting forceps are the tool of choice for cutting ribs and cracking the femur to extract bone marrow.

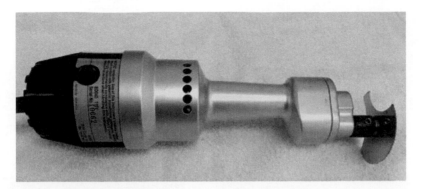

Figure 2.3 An oscillating saw (Figure 2.1e) is the most efficient way to cut the skull and remove the brain in dogs and cats. The saw can also be used to cut the dorsal lamina of the vertebral column to remove the spinal cord.

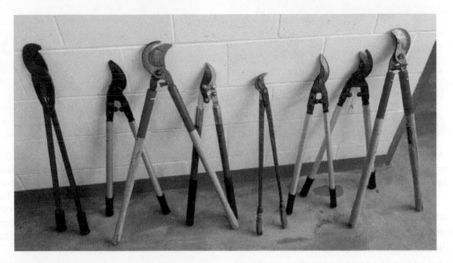

Figure 2.4 In large dogs, hedge clippers are often required to cut through the ribs and femur. These instruments are available in a variety of sizes and styles.

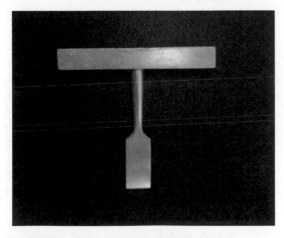

Figure 2.5 A T tool is used to loosen the top of the calvarium after the bone has been cut.

4) *Cutting board*

A standard synthetic kitchen cutting board provides a flat surface on which to section tissues and can be used as a background for photographs. Cutting tissues on the cutting board, rather than on a steel table, helps to keep your knife sharp. Wet tissues are often slippery. Covering the cutting board with a white paper towel (do not use colored paper towels as they can alter tissue color) will minimize slippage and allow for precise sections.

5) *Scale*

The body is always weighed prior to starting a necropsy, and most clinics and laboratories have a scale available for that purpose. Weights of organs, such as the heart and

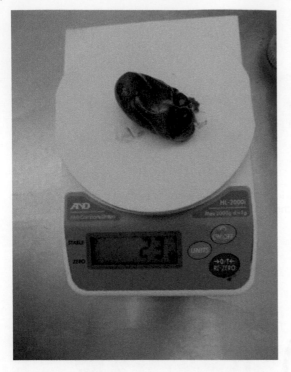

Figure 2.6 A gram scale is to determine body weight in small mammals, fetuses and newborn puppies and kittens, and to weigh organs.

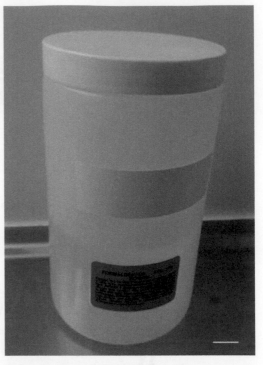

Figure 2.7 To collect samples for histopathology, use a wide-mouth container, containing 10% neutral buffered formalin. Initially fill only approximately one third of the container, to make the container bottom-heavy and less likely to spill, and to avoid overflow when tissues are added. Then, top off the container with formalin after the tissues are collected to achieve a final tissue to formalin ratio of 1:10. Scale bar = 2 cm.

liver, can also provide important information which may influence the diagnosis (Fig. 2.6). A smaller scale, with a range from 5 to 300 g, is a useful piece of equipment when performing a necropsy. These gram scales are available from a scientific supply company. Data for normal organ weights (as a percentage of body weight) are included in Appendix 1.

6) *Digital camera*

A digital camera is an amazing tool for recording and sharing findings from the necropsy examination; however, trying to keep the camera clean during the procedure can be difficult. At Cornell, we have a dedicated necropsy camera that remains on the necropsy floor at all times, and pictures are downloaded to a computer for access from our personal computers. Another option would be to invest in a relatively inexpensive waterproof case for your camera, tablet or smart phone. A camera with a resolution of at least 5 MP should be adequate for gross photography.

7) *Materials for collecting histopathology samples*

Samples which will be submitted for histopathology should be collected in a wide-mouth, plastic, leak-proof container (Fig. 2.7), with a final ratio of 1 part tissue to 10 parts fixative. The standard fixative is 10% neutral buffered formalin, which is available from any biological supply company. Other useful materials for collecting samples for histology include:

a) Wooden tongue depressors to affix samples of nerve, skin, and muscle to help maintain proper orientation during fixation.

b) Plastic tissue cassettes to differentiate lymph nodes, identify small tissues, or

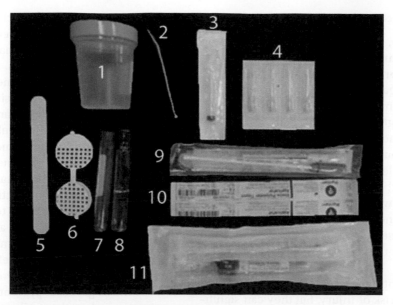

Figure 2.8 Supplies for collecting tissue for histopathology and ancillary testing: (1) Specimen cup for collecting feces or measuring effusions; (2) Zip tie to tie off a loop of bowel for ancillary testing; (3 and 4) Syringe and needles for collecting urine, blood, CSF, or synovial fluid. Can also be used to insufflate lungs and inject formalin into the gastrointestinal tract in small mammals; (5) Tongue depressor to affix skin, muscle, and nerve samples so they will fix flat for histopathology; (6) Red top tube for storing and transporting fluids for ancillary testing; and (7–10) Swabs and tubes for collecting samples for bacterial cultures.

mark specific lesions. If the tissue is small enough to be placed in a cassette without compression or crushing, do so. If not, clip the cassette to the edge of the tissue. Always label these cassettes with a #2 pencil; other types of markings will wash off in the formalin.

8) *Materials for collecting ancillary testing samples*

Always check with your diagnostic lab about instructions for submission of samples for ancillary tests, as the requirements may vary. In general, the following supplies will facilitate collection and submission of samples for the majority of diagnostic testing (Fig. 2.8):

a) Needles and syringes for collection of blood, urine, effusions, CSF, or synovial fluid
b) Red top blood tubes for storage and transport of collected fluids
c) Amies transport media (without charcoal) with swabs for aerobic cultures
d) BB™ Port-a-Cul™ or other anaerobic transport media with swabs
e) Plastic fecal cups to collect feces and stomach contents
f) String or zip ties to tie off loops of intestine
g) Small zipper lock bags to collect samples of individual organs for toxicology, virology, or bacteriologic testing.

2.3 Safety Considerations

The practice of veterinary medicine requires an assumption of risk and the necropsy is no exception. "Zero risk" is not achievable with biological systems, but knowledge of the risks associated with the necropsy can help keep the risk to an acceptable minimum. Knife cuts, punctures from hypodermic needles, exposure to formalin fumes, and exposure to zoonotic agents are the primary risks encountered in a small animal necropsy.

2.3.1 Cuts and Punctures

Unfortunately, cuts to the hands are a common necropsy injury. Prevention of cuts is best achieved by practice and use of a sharp knife. Dissecting a carcass with sharp implements is quick, efficient and allows for precise cuts. Sawing through tissues with a dull knife is tedious, impairs accurate dissection, and is potentially dangerous as excess force may cause the knife to slip leading to cut and stab injuries, especially to the hands. Most cuts occur late in the necropsy when fatigue leads to inattention. Ideally, the necropsy should be performed when the prosector is alert and well rested and not delegated to the end of a long and arduous day.

Cut-resistant gloves (Fig. 2.9) are one way to decrease the risk of injury, but they can significantly interfere with tactile sensation and dexterity. A reasonable compromise which we use in cases with known zoonotic potential is to just use one on the non-dominant hand. A great deal of confusion surrounds cut-resistant gloves. Cut-resistant gloves are generally rated on a scale of 1–5, but the standard used in the United States is based on the amount of weight needed to cut through a material when applied to a razor blade while the European standard counts the number of rotations needed for a circular

blade to cut through a material while moving laterally under a constant weight. Thus, two gloves with the same rating may have very different cut-resistant properties. Further, there is no requirement for North American manufacturers to certify the cut-resistance of their gloves. Cut-resistant gloves can be made from chain mesh, ultra-high molecular weight polyethylene, aramid fiber, fiber-metal blends, and combinations of layers, thicknesses, substrates and surface coatings. Importantly, while cut-resistant gloves provide protection from slashes by knives, they provide little to no protection from puncture wounds, such as a hypodermic needle. Cut-resistant gloves made from ultra-high molecular weight polyethylene provide excellent protection, can be worn between two latex or nitrile gloves to prevent body fluid contamination and can be sterilized and re-used.

Use of a scalpel incurs some additional risks. Scalpel blades dull rapidly necessitating frequent changes, and cuts often occur while the blade is being changed. Also, the tip of a scalpel blade can easily snap off within the tissue if the blade is twisted, creating a serious hazard. If this happens, use forceps or another instrument (not your fingers) to search for the blade. Not retrieving the blade can pose a risk to individuals handling the carcass during disposal.

2.3.2 Zoonotic Disease

Persons who are immunocompromised, immunosuppressed, on oral antibiotics or are pregnant are at increased risk of contracting a zoonotic disease. While transmission of a zoonotic disease during a necropsy is possible, the risk is less than in other areas of veterinary medical practice. A live animal can discharge infectious agents through body fluids throughout the environment, potentially exposing both animals and people. The microbiologist often works with a highly concentrated pure culture of a zoonotic agent. In contrast, if the necropsy is performed in a controlled environment with reasonable precautions, the risk of zoonotic disease transmission is very small.

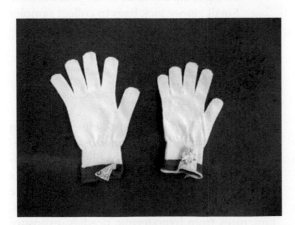

Figure 2.9 Cut resistant gloves can be used on the non-dominant hand. These gloves provide protection against accidental cuts and stab wounds.

Personal protective equipment (PPE) at a minimum includes latex exam gloves (ammonium nitrile gloves are an alternative if one has an allergy to latex). A pair of dedicated coveralls and an outer plastic apron will prevent contamination of work clothes. The plastic apron can be cleaned and disinfected with any standard disinfectant used to clean cages and work surfaces or disposable aprons can be used. The coveralls are best washed separately from work clothes using bleach. If a zoonotic disease is suspected, consider referring the case to a diagnostic laboratory, or, at a minimum, using additional PPE such as a respirator (surgeon's-type mask), splash shield and disposable coveralls.

2.3.3 Formalin

Formalin (10% formaldehyde) is the most common fixative used in pathology. Formaldehyde is a known human carcinogen (myeloid leukemia, sinonasal adenocarcinoma, and nasopharyngeal cancers). Acute exposure can cause skin and mucous membrane irritation. Formaldehyde is a sensitizing agent that can cause contact dermatitis (Type IV hypersensitivity) and anaphylactic reactions (Type I hypersensitivity). Contamination of cytologic preparations with formalin fumes will interfere with quick Wright–Giemsa-type stains (e.g., Diff-Quik® and Quick-Dip®). Thus, one should minimize exposure to formalin. Use of a wide mouth container with the lid screwed on a quarter turn will minimize fumes and make it easy to add tissues. A container that is only one-quarter to one-third full will be base heavy, making it harder to tip over and in the event of an accident, less formalin will spill. Small formalin spills (<100 ml) are best dealt with by absorbing the spilled material with paper towels. Place the paper towels in a labeled hazardous waste container, such as a heavy-duty plastic bag. Wash the contaminated area two or three times with soap and water and dry the area with paper towels. Place these paper towels in the labeled hazardous waste container,

seal it to minimize the release of formaldehyde vapors, and dispose of according to applicable state and local regulations. Larger spills are best handled using a commercial formaldehyde spill kit, available from a variety of manufacturers.

2.4 The Importance of a Good History

A thorough review of the medical record and clarification of the questions to be answered should be undertaken before beginning a necropsy. While some pathologists prefer to do a necropsy without prior knowledge of the medical history so that they are not biased, we strongly believe the necropsy should be guided by all available information. The medical review will highlight organ systems that may need extra attention and ensure the necessary supplies for collecting appropriate samples for ancillary tests are at hand before beginning the necropsy.

2.5 The Necropsy Report

The necropsy report is a way to convey your findings to a referring veterinarian, client, or pathologist who will be doing the histologic analysis of tissues. Pictures are a valuable addition to a necropsy report. A standard necropsy report is divided into four sections:

2.5.1 Gross Description

This is an objective account of all the gross lesions found during the necropsy examination. Usually the first sentence identifies the body and assesses the body condition and degree of postmortem autolysis:

> *Examined is the body of a 4.5kg, 4-year-old, female, spayed, brown Miniature Dachshund with a Purina body condition score of 5 out of 9 and mild postmortem autolysis.*

Evidence of medical manipulation is described, but postmortem artifacts are not. Also, normal findings are not usually included unless they are unexpected (i.e., a grossly normal liver in a cat with jaundice or an empty uterus in a dog reported to be pregnant). The goal of this section is to describe the gross changes, as completely as possible (location, size, number, color, consistency, demarcation, etc.) without interpretation, although sometimes interpretations are included parenthetically. Appendix 4 provides some suggestions for describing gross lesions.

2.5.2 Gross Findings

This section provides a summary of any lesions. Unlike the previous section, this part of the report does interpret lesions, although these interpretations are subject to modification based on additional data from histopathology and ancillary tests. The format we use at Cornell is described next:

2.5.2.1 Inflammatory Lesion

ORGAN: Severity (minimal, mild, moderate or severe), distribution (focal, multifocal, multifocal to coalescing, locally extensive, diffuse) chronicity (acute, subacute, chronic), exudate or cellular infiltrate (suppurative, hemorrhagic, necrotizing, lymphoplasmacytic), process (pneumonia, gastritis, meningitis, etc.)

LUNG: *Severe, acute, locally extensive, cranioventral, suppurative bronchopneumonia*

2.5.2.2 Effusion or Hemorrhage

LOCATION/ORGAN: Severity, descriptor, process

ABDOMINAL CAVITY: *Moderate hemorrhagic effusion*

2.5.2.3 Neoplasm, Congenital Defect

ORGAN: Name of condition

LIVER: *Hepatocellular carcinoma*

2.5.3 Gross Diagnosis

This section is the bottom line finding from the necropsy: the cause of death and, if euthanized, the reason for euthanasia. The gross diagnosis can be definitive, presumptive or open, based on the necropsy findings.

Euthanasia

Hemodynamic shock secondary to gastric dilation and volvulus

2.5.4 Comment

The final section of a gross report provides an opportunity for communication about the necropsy findings and what they mean. If additional tests are pending, those are listed in the comment:

The most significant gross finding in this case is segmental hemorrhagic enteritis affecting the middle one-third of the jejunum. This finding in an 8-week old kitten is highly suggestive of panleukopenia (feline parvovirus infection). Histopathology and virus isolation are pending.

2.6 Postmortem Changes

Postmortem degradation of tissue begins just minutes after an animal dies. The rate of degradation varies from case to case and organ to organ. Factors that increase the rate of degradation include high ambient temperature and humidity, thick hair coat or adipose layer, and fever or bacteremia prior to death. Ideally, necropsies would be performed within a few hours of the animal's death; unfortunately such efficiency is not always possible. If a necropsy is delayed more than a few hours, the body should be refrigerated or kept in a cooler with ice until the examination can be performed. Freezing should be avoided unless refrigeration is not available and the necropsy cannot be performed in the next 24 hours.

Postmortem decomposition involves two separate processes: autolysis, or tissue breakdown by lysosomal enzymes, and putrefaction, or tissue breakdown by bacteria, protozoa and fungi. The cellular mechanisms of autolysis mirror those of necrosis or cell death in a living organism. Loss of substrates required for ATP production (oxygen and glucose) and accumulation of waste products (carbon dioxide and nitrogenous wastes) lead to dysregulation of ion gradients and pH. This loss of cellular homeostasis results in membrane disruption, including the membranes of lysosomes. Rupture of lysosomes releases hydrolytic enzymes that degrade other cellular components. Lysosomal enzymes are found in all cells, but the concentration of lysosomes varies from tissue to tissue. The rate of autolysis is related to the lysosomal concentration in the tissue. Gastric mucosa and pancreas show rapid autolysis; kidney, liver, and heart have an intermediate autolytic rate; and fibrous connective tissue has a low rate of autolytic change. Examples of mild, moderate, and severe autolysis are illustrated in Fig. 2.10.

Cell rupture leads to loss of normal anatomic barriers (like the intestinal mucosa) and release of pigments such as hemoglobin and bile. The released hemoglobin and bile will stain tissues red and green, respectively, and the process is

(A)

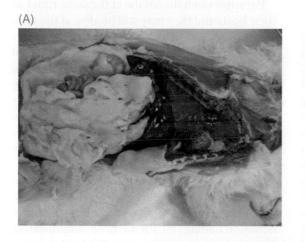

(B)

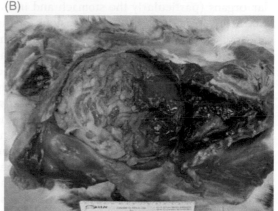

(C)

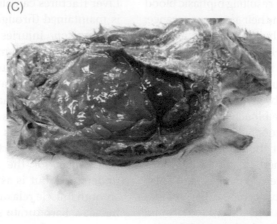

Figure 2.10 Degrees of postmortem decomposition. The cat in (A) shows mild postmortem changes, including bile staining of the omental fat and dark pink discoloration of the lungs. The cat in (B) shows moderate postmortem changes, including hemoglobin staining of the omental fat, black discoloration of the intestine (pseudomelanosis) secondary to the formation of iron sulfide and dark red to purple discoloration of the lungs. The puppy in (C) shows severe postmortem changes, including significant decomposition of the liver and dark green to black discoloration of the ventral abdominal body wall.

called hemoglobin or bile imbibition. The mixture of cytoplasm and degraded organelles is an excellent culture medium, and bacteria, protozoa, and fungi from the gastrointestinal tract, lungs, urinary tract, and skin begin to replicate and invade adjacent tissues. These organisms gradually break down tissues, and bacteria can produce hydrogen sulfide. Iron released from hemoglobin reacts with hydrogen sulfide produced by bacteria to form iron sulfide (FeS), which causes black discoloration of tissues (pseudomelanosis). Bacteria produce gas that creates an emphysematous change in solid organs and distention, or even rupture, of tubular organs (particularly the stomach and intestine). In some cases, the distension of the abdominal viscera can rupture the diaphragm and create a postmortem diaphragmatic hernia.

Other postmortem changes not directly related to decomposition include stiffening of the body (*rigor mortis*), cooling of the body (*algor mortis*) and the gravitational settling of blood in organs on the dependent side of a carcass (postmortem hypostasis or *livor mortis*). Often one lung, one kidney, even one half of the cerebral meninges will be darker red and sometimes the effect is dramatic. Also, the blood in the heart and large vessels will separate into plasma and cells, much as it does in a blood tube. The resulting biphasic blood clots are named based on their gross appearance: the plasma forms the "chicken fat clot" and the cells form the "currant jelly clot." The chicken fat clot is quite solid and can be mistaken for a tumor. Antemortem thrombi can be differentiated from postmortem blood clots by (1) presence of attachment to the intima of the blood vessel and/or (2) formation of discrete layers of blood cells ("lines of Zahn") indicating that the blood was flowing when the thrombus formed.

Agonal or perimortem changes are also common distractors in a necropsy. The sympathetic nervous system is often activated around the time of death, which can lead to rapid fluctuations in blood pressure and rupture of small blood vessels, such as those in the thymus and endocardium. The result is petechial or ecchymotic hemorrhages in these organs. Agonal breathing or variations in intrathoracic pressure around the time of death can cause some leakage of fluid into alveolar spaces. The fluid mixes with surfactant and forms foam, which is a common finding in the trachea and airways of cadavers. Animals with pulmonary edema will also have foamy fluid in the trachea and airways, but the lungs of an animal with pulmonary edema will be wet and heavy, and will exude fluid from the cut surface. A good test for pulmonary edema is to cut a section of the lung and set it aside. If after a few minutes, a puddle of fluid forms around the section, a diagnosis of pulmonary edema is warranted.

Parasites often do not die at the same times as their hosts and they may still be alive at the time of necropsy and/or may have migrated to aberrant locations. It is not unusual to see intestinal roundworms (typically ascarids) in the stomach, esophagus, or oral cavity in a cat or dog necropsy. Ectoparasites frequently outlive their hosts and may migrate to the nearest warm body, usually that of the prosector, during a necropsy. We keep a can of spray insecticide on the necropsy floor to help combat this problem.

Resuscitation efforts can cause a variety of changes that are evident during the necropsy. Cracked ribs and pulmonary contusions are common findings if CPR has been administered. Liver fractures can also occur. If blood pressure is maintained through the chest compressions, postmortem injuries will be associated with hemorrhage, which may lead to confusion since hemorrhage is often used as a sign that an injury occurred prior to death.

Barbiturate euthanasia is a common cause of postmortem changes that are misinterpreted as lesions. Barbiturates cause splenic congestion and enlargement, particularly in dogs. The exact mechanism for the phenomenon is not well understood, but is assumed to be secondary to smooth muscle relaxation in the capsule and trabeculae. Barbiturate salts can form precipitates on organ surfaces, especially in animals euthanized by intracardiac injection. These white crystals can be seen on the surface of the endocardium, pericardium, pleura, diaphragm, or even liver (Fig. 2.11). A large bolus of barbiturate

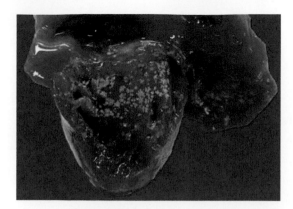

Figure 2.11 Barbiturate solution precipitate on the endocardial surface of the heart in a euthanized animal.

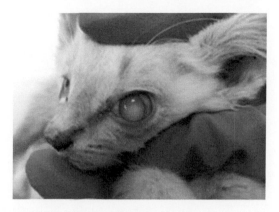

Figure 2.12 Opacity of the lens in a cat that was refrigerated after death (cold cataract).

euthanasia solution that reaches the right ventricle will lyse erythrocytes and convert the blood into a thick, red-brown pasty material. The material will have a characteristic "medicinal" or alcohol odor. Injection of barbiturate euthanasia solution outside the vasculature results in a chemical burn. Areas of brown discoloration are most noticeable in the lungs of animals euthanized by attempted intracardiac injection.

Changes that occur secondary to handling bodies after death include opacity of the ocular lens caused by cooling (also known as "cold cataracts"; Fig. 2.12). The lens opacity clears once the body warms up to room temperature. Accumulation of stomach contents in the nasal cavity can happen if a carcass is carried or hung with the head in a dependent position.

3

The Necropsy Procedure

3.1 Introduction

There are many ways to approach a necropsy (more than one way to skin and eviscerate a cat). The pages that follow describe one basic technique that is used at the Cornell College of Veterinary Medicine by pathologists, residents, and students. The technique borrows heavily from the ones described in *The Necropsy Book* by John King, et al. and *Necropsy Procedures and Basic Diagnostic Methods for Practicing Veterinarians* by Albert Strafuss. The technique presented is modified based on our insights gained by training pathology residents and teaching necropsy techniques to veterinary students. The procedure allows for inspection of all body regions and organs in such a way that no lesion should be overlooked while avoiding unnecessarily complex dissection schemes. The subsequent chapters break down the procedure by organ system and provide ideas for alternative techniques that may be useful based on the history or clinical findings in a particular case. For the most part, the sequence of the steps in a necropsy is not important, but we encourage using a standard procedure to ensure that all organs are examined and all samples collected. However, this procedure can be modified to accommodate specific circumstances. For example, if primary gastrointestinal disease is suspected, removal and examination of the intestines first is recommended due to the rapid rate of mucosal autolysis. Or, if pneumonia is suspected, the lungs should be removed and

sampled first in order to minimize the chances of cross contamination with gut flora.

3.2 Weigh the Body

Measuring and recording the body weight (Fig. 3.1) is an important first step in a necropsy for several reasons. One of the most important is to provide a basis for determining relative size of viscera. Particularly heart and brain weights are most useful when compared to the total body weight (see Appendix 1).

3.3 External Examination

The external examination is very similar to the physical examination of a living animal. The purpose of the external examination is to establish or confirm the identifying features of the animal (species, breed, sex, coat color, identifying markings, and tattoo or microchip number; Fig. 3.2), to document evidence of medical or surgical intervention and to detect and describe any external lesions. This step includes visual examination of the eyes, ears, oral cavity, skin and hair coat, nails, external genitalia, and perineum and palpation of the skull, limbs, joints, ribs, vertebrae, and pelvis. Note any discharges from body orifices. If the birth date is unknown, tooth eruption and wear patterns can be used to estimate the age of the animal (see Chapter 16). The retina can be

Necropsy Guide for Dogs, Cats, and Small Mammals, First Edition. Edited by Sean P. McDonough and Teresa Southard.
© 2017 John Wiley & Sons, Inc. Published 2017 by John Wiley & Sons, Inc.
Companion Website: www.wiley.com/go/mcdonough/necropsy

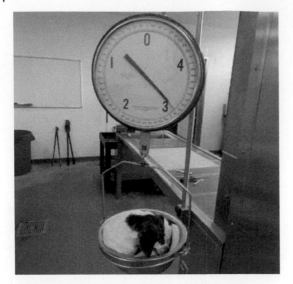

Figure 3.1 Before beginning the necropsy, weigh the body. Body weight provides objective information on body condition and is useful for determining atrophy or hypertrophy of organs judged to be abnormal in size.

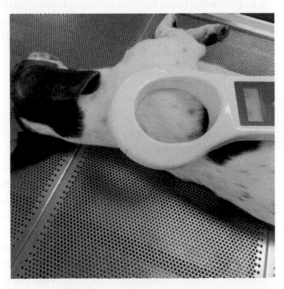

Figure 3.2 Before beginning the necropsy, document evidence of medical or surgical intervention and check for the presence of a microchip.

inspected by flattening the cornea with a glass microscope slide and shining a penlight through the pupil (see Chapter 12). Abdominal distention can be due to the accumulation of fat,

distention of the gastrointestinal tract with food or gas, accumulation of hemorrhage or ascitic fluid, or advanced pregnancy in female dogs and cats. Depending on the degree of rigor mortis, it may not be possible to palpate internal organs. Assessment and documentation of body condition score and degree of postmortem change provides useful data in cases where little history is available or the circumstances of the death are unknown. An overview photograph of the body as a whole (Fig. 3.3) and photographs of all external lesions should be taken before making the first incision.

3.4 Reflect the Skin and Right Limbs

Place the body in left lateral recumbency and begin with a stab incision in the right axilla (Fig. 3.4). This initial incision should be the only time the sharp edge of your knife contacts the haired side of the skin. To keep your knife sharp, additional skin incisions should be made by inserting the knife blade in the subcutis and cutting from the inside out. Extend the skin incision cranially along the mid line to the mandibular symphysis (Fig. 3.5) and caudally to the perineum, just dorsal to the external genitalia. In male dogs, incise the skin along either side of the prepuce and reflect the prepuce and penis caudally (Fig. 3.6). If the animal is an intact male with scrotal testes, remove the testes at this point by incising the scrotal skin and transecting the spermatic cord. Either leave a longer segment of spermatic cord attached to the left testes or make a small transverse nick in the right testis to help distinguish left from right.

Cut the pectoral muscles and brachial plexus to reflect the right forelimb. Locate the glenohumoral joint by depressing the forelimb, which will elevate the joint. Cut across the medial side of the joint at the highest point of the shoulder (Fig. 3.7). Assess the volume, color, and viscosity of synovial fluid (see Chapter 5). Inspect and palpate the articular cartilage and examine the joint capsule insertion line for irregularities

Figure 3.3 An overview photograph of the body and of all external lesions should be taken before making the first incision.

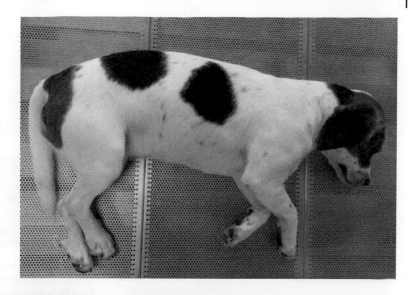

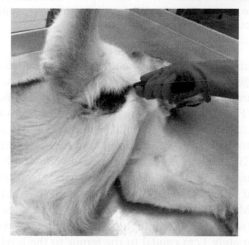

Figure 3.4 With the body in left lateral recumbency, begin with a stab incision in the right axilla. This should be the only time the sharp edge of your knife contacts the haired side of the skin.

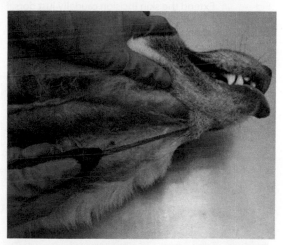

Figure 3.5 Extend the skin incision in the axilla cranially along the mid line to the mandibular symphysis.

that might indicate new bone growth due to osteoarthritis. Evaluate the synovial lining and the thickness of the fibrous layer of the joint capsule.

Reflect the skin dorsally to expose the thoracic and abdominal wall from the ventral midline to the level of the vertebral transverse processes. In adult females, examine the mammary gland tissue as you reflect the skin and collect samples

of any nodules or areas of thickening, as well as a section of normal gland.

Palpate the coxofemoral junction to locate the joint space and open the joint capsule. In small or thin animals, it is very easy to accidently cut into the abdominal cavity as you are opening the coxofemoral joint, so angle the knife away from the body wall. Cut the ligament of the head of the femur (Fig. 3.8) and the surrounding musculature to reflect the right hind limb dorsally. Examine the joint. Next reflect the skin

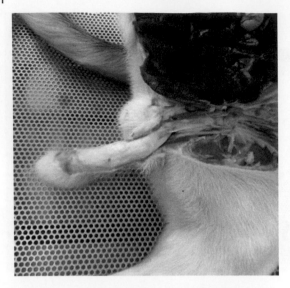

Figure 3.6 Extend the skin incision caudally just dorsal to the external genitalia. In male dogs reflect the prepuce and penis caudally. If the animal is an intact male with scrotal testes, incise the scrotal skin and transect the spermatic cord to collect the testes.

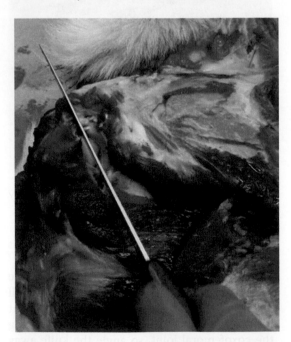

Figure 3.7 Opening the glenohumoral joint is facilitated by depressing the forelimb. Cut on the medial side over the highest point to enter the joint cavity. Note the appearance of the articular cartilage, synovial fluid, joint capsule, and the presence of any periarticular osteophytes.

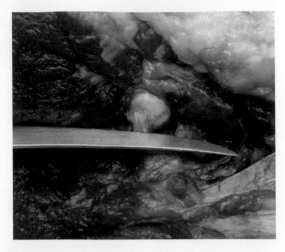

Figure 3.8 Cut the ligament of the head of the femur and the surrounding musculature to reflect the right hind limb dorsally. When opening the coxofemoral joint in small or thin animals, take care not to inadvertently puncture the abdominal cavity.

past the stifle and open the knee joint. This is best accomplished by flexing the joint and making a transverse cut in the patellar ligament (Fig. 3.9). Insert the tip of the knife next to the medial trochlea (Fig. 3.10) and incise the soft tissues to reflect the patella laterally (Fig. 3.11). Transect the lateral and medial collateral ligaments. Visualization of the menisci is facilitated if the cruciate ligaments are cut (Fig. 2.12). Make a cut through the medial thigh muscles (sartorius and adductor) parallel and approximately 1 cm caudal to the femur to the level of the medial aspect of the biceps femoris muscle to expose the sciatic nerve (Fig. 3.13). Collect a section of sciatic nerve, skeletal muscle, and skin, and affix these samples to a wooden tongue depressor or piece of cardboard (Fig. 3.14). Allow the tissue to dry for 1–2 minutes and put the tongue depressor with attached tissues into the fixative jar (be sure the tissues are completely submerged). Clear the skeletal muscle away from the proximal end of the femur and use bone forceps or hedge clippers to make an angled cut through the metaphysis. The diagonal cut usually causes a comminuted break in the bone, allowing for collection of

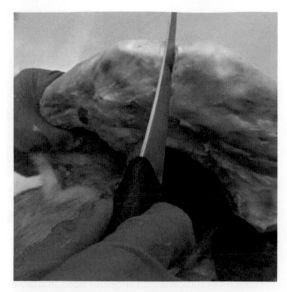

Figure 3.9 After reflecting the skin away from the stifle, flex the knee joint and make a transverse cut through the middle of the patellar ligament. Extend the incision medially and laterally to incise the collateral ligaments.

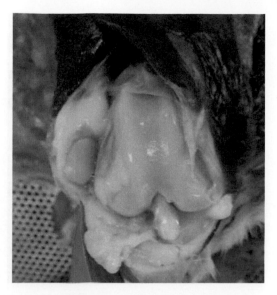

Figure 3.11 Reflect the patella laterally to inspect the cruciate ligaments and menisci.

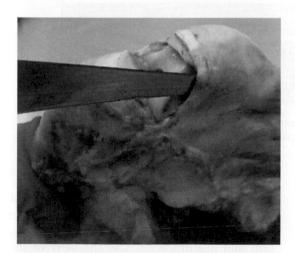

Figure 3.10 To reflect the patella, insert the tip of the knife next to the medial trochlea and incise the soft tissues.

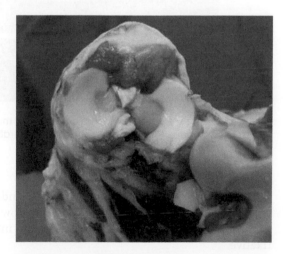

Figure 3.12 Visualization of the menisci is facilitated if the cruciate ligaments are cut.

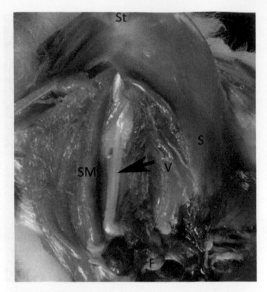

Figure 3.13 To collect a section of sciatic nerve, make a cut along the medial aspect of the thigh, parallel and caudal to the femur. Femoral head (F), stifle (St), sartorius muscle (S), vastus medialis muscle (V), and semimembranosus muscle (SM).

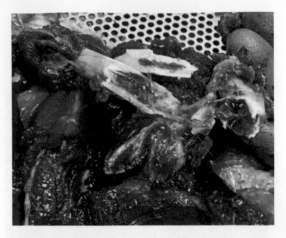

Figure 3.15 A diagonal cut with rib cutters across the proximal femoral diaphysis usually causes a comminuted break in the bone, allowing for collection of samples of cortical bone, cancellous bone, and bone marrow. Place the bone marrow in a labelled tissue cassette and immerse in fixative.

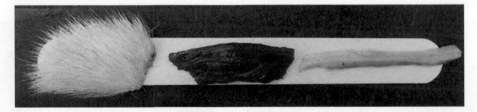

Figure 3.14 Collect a section of sciatic nerve, skeletal muscle, and skin. To ensure proper orientation, affix these samples to a wooden tongue depressor or piece of cardboard, allow the samples to adhere for 1–2 min and then place in fixative.

samples of cortical bone, cancellous bone and bone marrow (Fig. 3.15). Place the bone marrow in a labelled tissue cassette and immerse in fixative.

3.5 Open the Abdominal Cavity

The next step is to open the abdominal cavity by cutting through the abdominal wall to create a flap that is reflected ventrally. The initial cut should be made just caudal to the costal arch at the highest point of the abdomen. By cutting at the highest point, any fluid within the abdomen can be retained in the cavity, allowing for collection and quantification. Use the belly of the blade and make a 4–5 cm incision through each muscle plane and the peritoneum. Once you have entered the abdominal cavity elevate the body wall to help prevent inadvertently incising the underlying viscera (Fig. 3.16). Extend the incision along the costal arch ventrally to the xiphoid process, dorsally to the lumbar vertebral muscles (longissimus), caudally to the ilium, and ventrally as close to the pubic bones as possible. (Fig. 3.17).

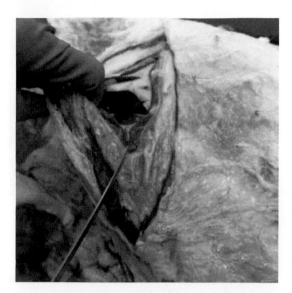

Figure 3.16 To open the abdomen, make the initial cut just caudal to the costal arch at the highest point and then elevate the body wall to help prevent inadvertently incising the underlying viscera.

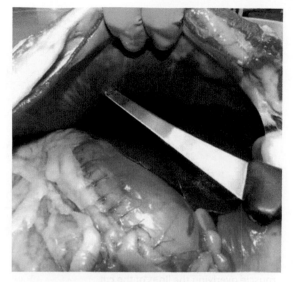

Figure 3.18 Puncture the diaphragm at the highest point, near the insertion onto the last rib and listen for an inrush of air indicating negative pressure in the thorax. Once the diaphragm has been cut, the muscle should flatten out and become flaccid.

3.6 Puncture the Diaphragm

Once the abdomen is open, observe the shape of the diaphragm. The muscle should be taut and concave. Use your blade to cut through the diaphragm at the highest point, near the insertion onto the last rib (again, aim for the highest point to retain any fluid in the thoracic cavity). Once the diaphragm has been cut, the muscle should flatten out and become flaccid (Fig. 3.18). In a very fresh cadaver, you may hear a rush of air into the thoracic cavity. With prolonged postmortem intervals, negative pressure will often be lost. Once negative thoracic pressure has been assessed, use your blade to cut through the entire right side of the diaphragm as close as possible to the costal arch.

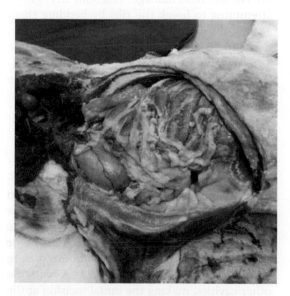

Figure 3.17 Extend the initial abdominal incision along the costal arch ventrally to the xiphoid process, dorsally to the lumbar vertebral muscles (longissimus), caudally to the ilium, and ventrally as close to the pubic bones as possible to create a flap that is reflected ventrally.

3.7 Open the Thoracic Cavity

In heavily muscled dogs, it is helpful to incise the muscle overlying the lines of the cut (Fig. 3.19). Opening the thoracic cavity involves

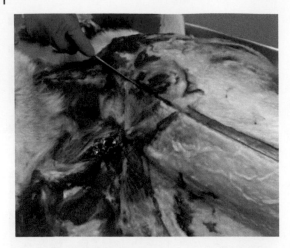

Figure 3.19 To open the thoracic cavity, cut the ribs. In heavily muscled dogs, it is helpful to incise the muscle overlying the lines of the cut.

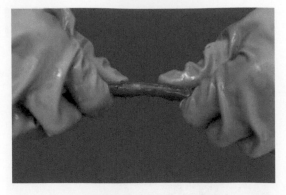

Figure 3.21 Test bone strength by attempting to break the ribs by bending them against the curvature. If they break, they should snap crisply.

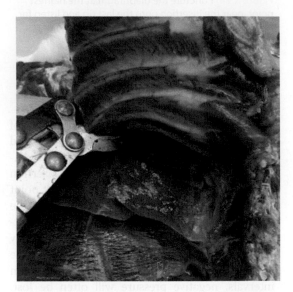

Figure 3.20 To enter the thoracic cavity, make two cuts through the rib cage. First cut though the cartilaginous attachments of the ribs to the sternum, then through the dorsal aspect of the ribs, slightly ventral to the articulation with the vertebral transverse processes. Using your non-dominant hand to retract the thoracic wall as you go helps to visualize the viscera and avoid damage.

making two cuts through the rib cage: one though the cartilaginous attachments of ribs to the sternum and one through the dorsal aspect

of the ribs, slightly ventral to the articulation with the vertebral transverse processes (Fig. 3.20). In young animals, the cut adjacent to the sternum can be made with a knife or scalpel; however, bone forceps or hedge clippers are needed to cut through the dorsal aspects of the ribs. Using your non-dominant hand to retract the thoracic wall as you go helps to visualize the viscera and avoid damage. Test bone strength by attempting to break the ribs by bending them against the curvature (Fig. 3.21). If they break, they should snap crisply. In young animals, free a central rib and check the costochondral junction by cutting along the cranial edge (See Fig. 5.7).

3.8 Open the Pericardium

The third body cavity to open is the pericardium. In a normal animal, this thin sac is in close apposition to the epicardium and can be difficult to grasp or cut without damaging the underlying heart. Using rat tooth forceps or your fingers to tent the pericardium before incising it may be helpful (Fig. 3.22). As with the other cavities, making the initial incision at the highest point is helpful for retaining any effusion for quantification. In a cat or dog, the pericardium typically contains about 0.25 ml/kg of thin, clear, translucent to straw colored fluid. Reflect

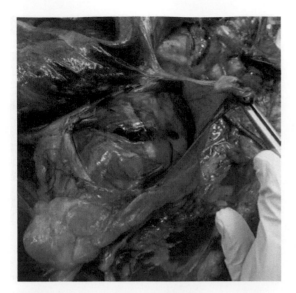

Figure 3.22 To open the pericardium without slicing into the underlying heart, use rat tooth forceps or fingers to tent the pericardium before incising it. In a cat or dog, the pericardium typically contains about 0.25 ml/kg of thin, clear, translucent to straw colored fluid.

3.9 *In Situ* Examination of Organs

Once all three body cavities have been opened, the organs should be examined *in situ*. Note the position and color of the organs, the characteristics of any fluid in the thorax, abdomen or pericardial sac and assess the degree of autolysis. Sometimes the hardest lesion to recognize is a missing organ, so check for the presence or absence of both kidneys, the spleen, the female reproductive tract, and the adrenals. This pause in the procedure provides a great opportunity for an overview photo (Fig. 3.24). Some gross diagnoses, such as an extrahepatic shunt, an obstructed bile duct, or an intestinal displacement, can only be fully appreciated with the organs still intact. Remove and inspect the omentum (Fig. 3.25) to allow full visualization of the abdominal organs. The left kidney and adrenal gland can be visualized by reflecting the intestines dorsally.

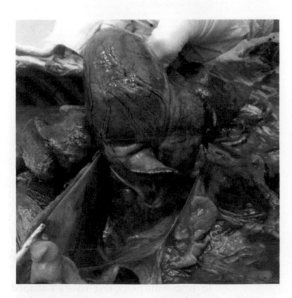

Figure 3.23 Reflect the apex of the heart dorsally to inspect the lining of the pericardial sac and the pulmonary veins returning to the left atrium.

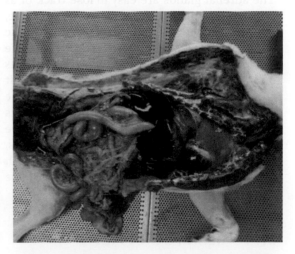

Figure 3.24 Once all three body cavities have been opened (thorax, abdomen, and pericardial sac), the organs should be examined *in situ*. Note the position and color of the organs, the characteristics of any fluid, and assess the degree of autolysis. An overview photograph is useful at this point to refresh your memory when writing the necropsy report.

the apex of the heart dorsally to inspect the lining of the pericardial sac and the pulmonary veins returning to the left atrium (Fig. 3.23).

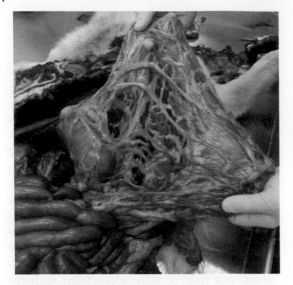

Figure 3.25 Remove and inspect the omentum to allow full visualization of the small intestine.

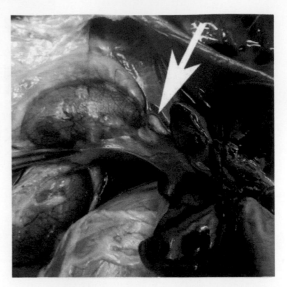

Figure 3.26 The first organs harvested should be the adrenal glands since they are easily overlooked as other abdominal viscera are removed. The adrenal glands lie just cranial to the kidneys (white arrow) and the caudal pole is usually embedded in fat.

3.10 Remove the Adrenal Glands

The adrenal glands are easy to lose track of as other abdominal viscera are removed; therefore, we recommend finding and collecting these organs first (Fig. 3.26). The adrenal glands lie just cranial to kidneys and the caudal pole is often embedded in fat. To visualize the left adrenal gland it is often necessary to reflect the intestine dorsally. Locating the adrenal glands is easy in young, thin, fresh carcasses, but can be quite difficult in obese, autolyzed carcasses, especially those with a history of treatment with exogenous corticosteroids. (see Chapter 13: The Endocrine System).

3.11 Remove the Pluck

The oral, cervical, and thoracic viscera, including the tongue, larynx, esophagus, trachea, thyroid and parathyroid glands, thymus, lungs, and heart, are removed as a unit (the pluck). The first step is to make a V-shaped incision along the medial aspect of the body of both mandibles

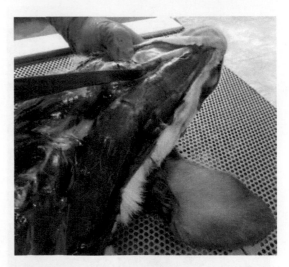

Figure 3.27 To remove the pluck, first make a V-shaped incision along the medial aspect of the body of both mandibles from the ramus to the mandibular symphysis.

from the ramus to the mandibular symphysis (Fig. 3.27). Cut through the frenulum that attaches the base of the tongue to the oral mucosa (Fig. 3.28) and extract the tongue ventrally

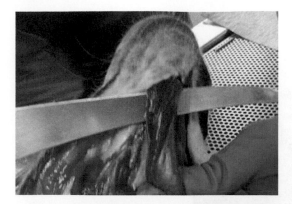

Figure 3.28 Cut through the frenulum that attaches the base of the tongue to the oral mucosa and extract the tongue ventrally through the intermandibular space.

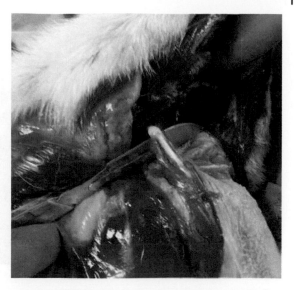

Figure 3.30 At the level of the angle of the mandible, the hyoid apparatus must be cut through the synchondrosis between the epihyoid and stylohyoid bones. In most small animals the cartilage can be cut with a scalpel blade. On occasion, the joint is fused with bone and will need to be cut with a pair of bone forceps.

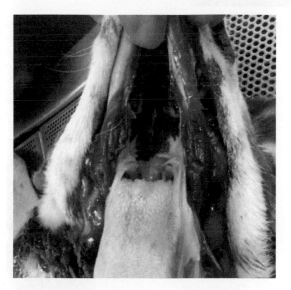

Figure 3.29 Grasp the tongue and reflect it caudally while cutting the oropharyngeal tissues. As the soft palate is transected cranially and laterally to the epiglottis, inspect the tonsils.

through the intermandibular space. If the tongue is trapped between the teeth due to rigor mortis, insert a sturdy pair of scissors or the steel behind the canine teeth and pry the jaws open. If this fails to free the tongue, cut the mandibular symphysis with rib cutters or a saw and spread the two mandibles apart.

Grasp the tongue and reflect it caudally while cutting the oropharyngeal tissues. For a better view of the oral cavity, remove one of the mandibles after the pluck has been harvested (see Chapter 8: The Alimentary System). As the soft palate is transected cranially and laterally to the epiglottis, inspect the tonsils (Fig. 3.29). At the level of the angle of the mandible, the hyoid apparatus must be cut. Palpate for and cut through the synchondrosis between the epihyoid and stylohyoid bones (Fig. 3.30; also see Fig. 5.4). After disarticulating the hyoid bones, continue to reflect the tongue, larynx, trachea and esophagus to the thoracic inlet, taking care to keep the thyroid glands with the pluck. Examine the jugular veins, vagus nerves, and carotid arteries as you dissect out the cranial part of the pluck. At the thoracic inlet, cut the vessels to the forelimb and then sever the sternopericaridial ligament (Fig. 3.31) that extends between the pericardium and sternum and reflect the aorta from the thoracic vertebral column (Fig. 3.32). Finally, transect the aorta (Fig. 3.33), caudal vena cava (Fig. 3.33), and esophagus (Fig. 3.34) to remove the pluck from the thoracic cavity (Fig. 3.35).

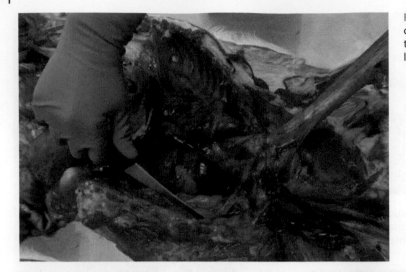

Figure 3.31 At the thoracic inlet, cut the vessels to the forelimb and then sever the sternopericaridial ligament.

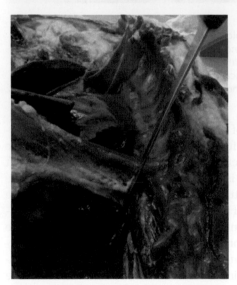

Figure 3.32 Continue to remove the pluck from the thoracic cavity by separating the aorta from the body wall.

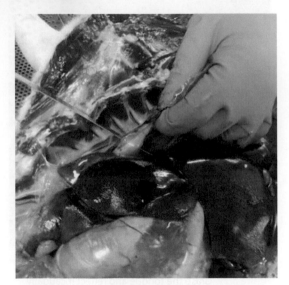

Figure 3.33 Next, transect the aorta and vena cava.

3.12 Remove the Gastrointestinal Tract, Liver, and Spleen

Before removing the abdominal organs, check the patency of the bile duct by squeezing the gall bladder and watching for a subtle distension of the distal duodenum. If no distension is detected, you can also make a small incision into the duodenum at the level of the bile duct insertion and look for the influx of bile (see Chapter 9: The Liver and Pancreas).

The easiest way to begin removing the abdominal organs is to first linearize the small intestine by incising the mesentery (Fig. 3.36). This allows for visual inspection and palpation of the entire small intestine. Next, locate and transect the rectum (Fig. 3.37). To avoid fecal contamination

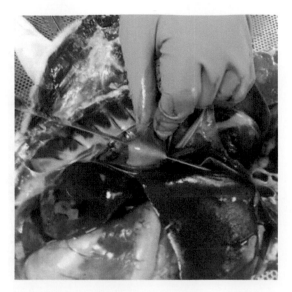

Figure 3.34 Finally, transect the esophagus and pull the organ block from the thoracic cavity.

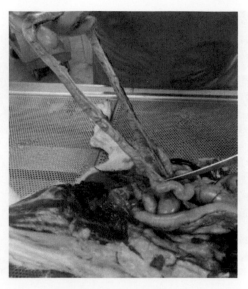

Figure 3.36 The first step in removing the abdominal viscera is to linearize the small intestine by cutting the mesentery. This allows for inspection and palpation of the entire length.

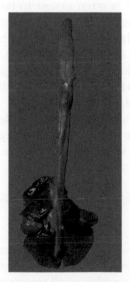

Figure 3.35 The excised pluck, including the tongue, trachea, esophagus, thyroid glands, thymus, heart, and lungs.

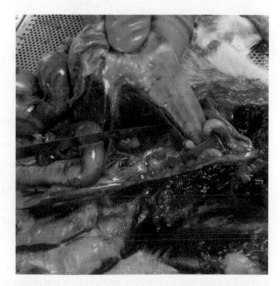

Figure 3.37 To avoid fecal contamination of the abdominal cavity when transecting the rectum, either milk the fecal material away from the site of transection or tie off the rectum with two pieces of string or two zip ties and cut between them. Once the rectum is transected, cut the mesocolon to the root of the mesentery.

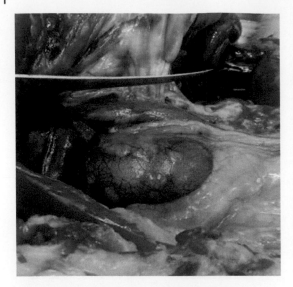

Figure 3.38 Incise the root of the mesentery. The kidneys should remain in the body cavity as you remove the alimentary tract, but it is often easiest to take the spleen, pancreas, and liver with attached diaphragm out with the digestive tract.

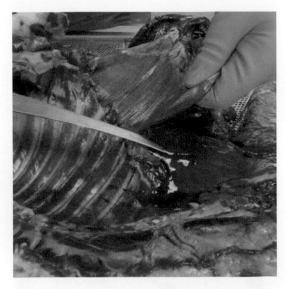

Figure 3.39 Cut the diaphragm along its costal margin leaving it attached to the liver, to complete the removal of the alimentary tract.

of the abdominal cavity, either milk the fecal material away from the site of transection or tie off the rectum with two pieces of string or two zip ties and cut between them. Once the rectum

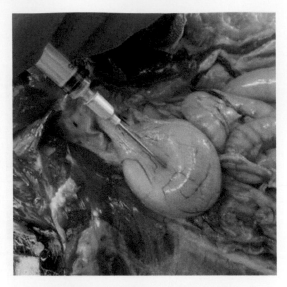

Figure 3.40 If desired, use a needle and syringe to collect a urine sample before removing the genitourinary tract.

is transected, cut the mesocolon to the root of the mesentery. The kidneys should remain in the body cavity as you remove the alimentary tract, but it is often easiest to take the spleen, pancreas and liver with attached diaphragm out with the digestive tract. Incise the root of the mesentery (Fig. 3.38) and then cut the diaphragm along its costal margin leaving it attached to the liver, to complete the removal of the alimentary tract (Fig. 3.39). Alternatively, you can incise the hepatoduodenal ligament and remove the liver and diaphragm separately. The spleen will come out with the stomach.

3.13 Remove the Urogenital Organs

If not already done, incise the scrotal skin of intact males and harvest the testes. Mark the right kidney with a small transverse incision so that the left and right kidneys can be distinguished once they are removed from the body. If desired, use a needle and syringe to collect a urine sample before removing the genitourinary tract (Fig. 3.40). Remove the genitourinary tract as a unit by incising the renal vessels and

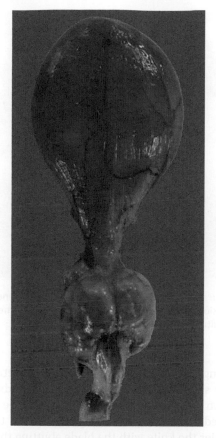

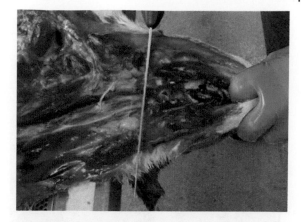

Figure 3.42 Disarticulate the atlanto-occipital joint. This is facilitated by inserting an index finger into the intermandibular space and hyperextending the head over the edge of the table.

Figure 3.41 After reflecting the kidneys and ureters to the urinary bladder, transect the urethra. In male animals cut the urethra caudal to the prostate gland.

then cutting anteriorly and laterally to the kidney to reflect the kidneys and ureters to the urinary bladder. In male animals, transect the urethra caudal to the prostate gland (Fig. 3.41). Chapter 10 describes a more advanced technique for splitting the pelvis to remove the entire genitourinary tract.

3.14 Remove the Head

Before removing the head, cerebrospinal fluid can be collected (if desired) via the traditional dorsal approach to the cisterna magna at the base of the skull. This is an excellent opportunity to practice this procedure. Alternatively, CSF can be collected via a ventral approach as described next. The head is disarticulated at the atlanto-occipital joint, a "V" shaped joint which is palpated by placing your fingers on the cranial ventral neck and extending and flexing the head (the "yes" joint). In brachycephalic dogs, the atlanto-occipital joint is often more rostral than one might expect. Cut through the muscles overlying the joint to expose the atlanto-occipital membrane. This is facilitated by inserting an index finger into the intermandibular space and hyperextending the head over the edge of the table (Fig. 3.42). CSF can be collected at this point by inserting a needle through the membrane (Fig. 3.43). Extend the neck and insert the point of your blade into the joint space to transect the spinal cord and the ligaments joining the atlas and occipital condyles (Fig. 3.44). Use manual pressure to further extend the neck while cutting the dorsal neck muscles and the skin to remove the head.

3.15 Take Out the Eyes

The most difficult part of removing the eyes is cutting the optic nerve and extraocular muscles in the retrobulbar space without accidentally puncturing the globe. A simple technique that helps to reduce the chance of puncturing the globe is to make a generous circumferential

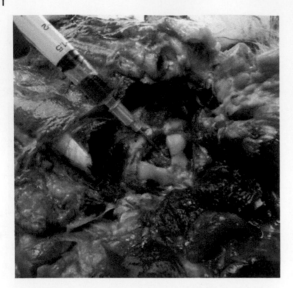

Figure 3.43 Cerebral spinal fluid can be collected by inserting a needle through the atlanto-occipital membrane.

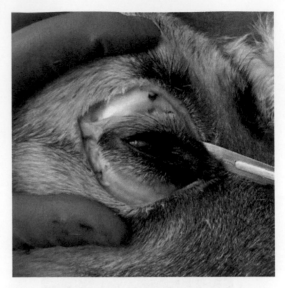

Figure 3.45 To remove the eyes, first make a generous incision in the skin around the eyelids and use the resulting flap as a handle to provide traction.

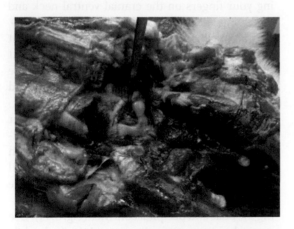

Figure 3.44 Extend the neck and insert the point of the blade into the joint space to transect the spinal cord and the ligaments joining the atlas and occipital condyles. Hyperextend the neck as the dorsal neck muscles and the skin are incised to complete removal of the head.

incision in the skin around the eyelids and use the eyelids as a handle to provide traction (Fig. 3.45). Using forceps or your hand to grasp the eyelid, insert your knife or scalpel blade

along the edge of the orbit to reach the retrobulbar structures. Once the eye and eyelids have been removed, excess soft tissue can be separated from the globe by pinching the tissues under the knife with the blade abutting the cornea but with the cutting edge angled slightly away so as to prevent inadvertent incisions. Gently pull the soft tissues back and forth under the knife with a moderate amount of traction. As the tissues are cut, the globe will begin to rotate. Watch carefully to prevent excision of the optic nerve. See Chapter 12 for more details on harvesting eyes.

3.16 Remove the Brain

Removal of the brain is perhaps the most difficult part of the necropsy, because the brain tissue is so soft and so intimately encased in the bony cranium. The best approach is to first reflect the skin from the head, by making a dorsal midline incision and reflecting the skin laterally. Then remove as much soft tissue from the skull as possible. Use either an

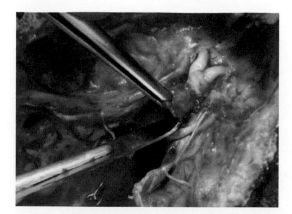

Figure 3.46 After removing the brain, transect the clinoid process caudal to the pituitary gland to provide better access. Gently grasp the meninges and gently dissect the pituitary from its attachments to the basisphenoid bone.

oscillating saw or bone cutters (depending on the size of the animal and your tolerance for damage to the brain) to cut the bone of the calvarium. Begin at the foramen magnum and make bilateral cuts along the dorsolateral aspect of the cranium (see Fig. 11.2–11.4). The initial cuts from the foramen magnum should be just medial to the occipital condyles and at a 45° angle from midline. Extend these cuts toward the orbits bilaterally, with a transverse cut connecting the two lateral cuts just caudal to the orbit.

The spinal cord is not routinely collected unless clinical signs indicate spinal cord disease. The techniques for removing the brain and spinal cord are described in detail in Chapter 11.

3.17 Remove the Pituitary Gland

The pituitary gland is discretely tucked away in the hypophyseal fossa (sella turcica) and is easily forgotten during a necropsy. Locate the gland just caudal to the optic chiasm. Use bone forceps or sturdy scissors to cut through the bone (posterior clinoid process of the sphenoid bone) caudal to and on both sides of the gland (see Chapter 13: The Endocrine System). Carefully grab the meninges adjacent to the gland with forceps and elevate the gland, using a scalpel blade, to carefully dissect the gland from the basisphenoid bone (Fig. 3.46). Because of the small size of the gland, it should be placed in a labeled cassette if submitting tissues for histopathology.

At this point, all organs have been removed. The next part of the necropsy involves careful examination of the organs and collection of samples for additional testing. Those steps are described in detail for each organ system in the chapters that follow.

Bibliography

King, John M, Roth-Johnson L, Newson, ME. 2007. *The Necropsy Book: A Guide for Veterinary Students, Residents, Clinicians, Pathologists, and Biological Researchers.* 5th edn. Gurnee, Ill.: Charles Louis Davis, DVM Foundation.

Strafuss, Albert C. 1988. *Necropsy Procedures and Basic Diagnostic Methods for Practicing Veterinarians.* Springfield, Ill: Charles C. Thomas, publisher.

Part II

Organ Systems

4

The Integumentary System

Necropsy examination of the integumentary system is very similar to dermatologic examination of a living animal, except that the patient is much more cooperative. The vocabulary of dermatology and dermatopathology is specialized, and a working knowledge of this vocabulary allows a prosector to effectively interpret and communicate necropsy findings.

4.1 Anatomy Review

The integument is composed of epidermis, dermis, adnexal structures, arrector pili muscles, and the subcutis. The adnexal structures, also known as pilosebaceous units, are composed of hair follicles, epitrichial sweat glands, and sebaceous glands. The mammary glands and apocrine glands of the anal sac are modified adnexal glands. Specialized structures such as claws, paw pads, nasal planum and external ear canals are also considered part of the integument.

Although the architecture of the skin is conserved across most mammalian species, there are differences between species and site differences within the same species. Most of the mammalian species discussed in this book are covered by hair. Exceptions include hairless breeds of dogs (i.e., Mexican hairless dog, Chinese crested dogs), cats (i.e., Sphynx cat), and small mammals such as the nude mouse. Microscopically these animals have hair follicles but their hair follicles are abnormal and are not able to produce normal hairs. Hairs that do form are usually fragile and break off as soon as they enter the infundibulum.

The dermis contributes most to the thickness of the skin. The haired skin is thickest over the dorsal surface of the body and lateral aspect of the limbs and thinnest on the ventral aspect of the trunk and medial limbs. In areas that lack hair such as the paw pads, nasal planum, and lips, the epidermis is thickest to protect from surface trauma. The epidermis is thinnest in well protected sites such as the ventral abdomen and inguinal areas. It is important to keep these differences in mind when taking skin samples for histologic evaluation. For example, if an endocrinopathy or negative energy balance, and thus atrophic dermatopathy, is suspected, the ventral abdomen and inguinal regions are not the preferred sampling sites since the skin is normally quite thin in these areas.

Hair serves a number of functions, including protection, thermal insulation, social communication, and sensory perception. Arrangement and type of hair follicles vary with species, breed, individual, and body region. However, in general, hair follicle density is greatest over the dorsolateral aspect of the body and least on the ventral aspect. Hair follicles are formed by a downward invagination of the surface ectoderm and are essentially an infolding of the epidermis. Hair follicles are classified as primary or secondary and simple or compound. Dogs, cats, rabbits, and ferrets have compound hair follicles; this gives them their dense coats. Plush coated arctic breeds have more secondary hairs

Necropsy Guide for Dogs, Cats, and Small Mammals, First Edition. Edited by Sean P. McDonough and Teresa Southard.
© 2017 John Wiley & Sons, Inc. Published 2017 by John Wiley & Sons, Inc.
Companion Website: www.wiley.com/go/mcdonough/necropsy

than breeds with coarser coats such as Labrador retrievers and Boxer dogs. Mice and rats have simple hair follicles. The pilosebaceous unit of a compound hair follicle is composed of one or more primary hair follicles surrounded by multiple secondary hair follicles. Primary hair follicles have a larger diameter, are embedded more deeply in the dermis or subcutis, and are associated with sebaceous and epitrichial sweat glands and an arrector pili muscle. Secondary hair follicles are smaller in diameter, are more superficial in the dermis, and may be accompanied by a sebaceous gland but lack a sweat gland and arrector pili muscle. Each hair of the compound follicle has its own papilla, but at the level of the sebaceous gland opening, the follicles unite to exit from a single external follicular orifice.

4.1.1 External Ear Canal Anatomy

In domestic animals, the pinnae are composed of flattened sheets of elastic cartilage covered by haired skin. Depending on the species or breed, pinnae may be erect or semi-erect, floppy or lop (Cocker Spaniels, Lop-eared rabbits), or folded (Scottish fold cats). Supportive elastic cartilage forms various folds that include the tragus, antitragus, helix, antihelix, and the marginal pouch (Henry's pouch; see Fig. 12.11) as part of the conical opening to the external auditory meatus (EAM). This canal gradually narrows with structural support from auricular and annular cartilage and merges into the osseous acoustic meatus. A complex group of skeletal muscles control pinnal movements. They are all innervated by the facial nerve. A unilateral drooping ear may be an indication of facial nerve paralysis.

Haired skin covers the convex and concave surface of the pinnae. Hair follicle numbers within the external ear canal decrease toward the tympanic membrane. In dogs, ceruminous glands, specialized apocrine glands, are more numerous near the tympanic membrane and decrease in number proximally as they move up the external ear canal. The density of sebaceous glands is the opposite: denser near the external

acoustic meatus and less dense near the tympanic membrane. The external surface of the tympanic membrane is covered by a thin layer of squamous epithelium that overlays a thin stromal layer containing blood vessels only in the stria mallearis adjacent to the manubrium of the malleus.

4.2 *In Situ* Examination and Removal

The skin, hair coat, nasal planum, paw pads, claws, and external ear canal should be thoroughly examined and all lesions should be sampled. Skin lesions are divided into primary lesions, which are directly related to the disease process, and secondary lesions, which either evolve from the primary lesions or are caused by external forces such as scratching, trauma, infection, or the healing process. The distinction between primary and secondary skin lesions is not always clear.

4.2.1 Primary Lesions

1) A macule is a circumscribed flat area of color change less than 1 cm in diameter. The color change may be hyperpigmentation such as in the black macules seen in lentigo simplex in orange cats or they may be hypopigmented macules as in vitiligo. A patch is essentially a large macule; a circumscribed flat area of color change that is greater than 1 cm in diameter.
2) A papule is a solid, elevated lesion, less than 1 cm in diameter. Papules can be follicular (i.e., staphylococcal folliculitis) or non-follicular (i.e., flea bite hypersensitivity). A nodule is a circumscribed solid elevation >1 cm in diameter that usually extends into deeper layers of skin.
3) A plaque is a less than 1 cm, slightly elevated, flat topped, and steep-walled lesion in skin. A feline eosinophilic plaque is a good example of a plaque.
4) A pustule is a circumscribed elevation of skin containing pus and therefore usually has

a white or pale yellow to green appearance. Like papules, pustules can be follicular (i.e., staphylococcal folliculitis) or non-follicular (i.e., pemphigus foliaceous).

5) A vesicle is a less than 1 cm, sharply circumscribed elevation of epidermis filled with clear fluid. Vesicles can be intraepidermal or subepidermal. A bulla is essentially a large vesicle. It is a collection of fluid within or below the epidermis that is sharply circumscribed and greater than 1 cm in diameter.

6) A wheal (i.e., urticaria) is a sharply circumscribed raised elevation in the skin consisting of edema. Wheals pit with pressure and are often erythematous.

7) A cyst is an epithelium-lined cavity containing fluid or a solid material. It is a smooth, well-circumscribed, fluctuant to solid mass.

4.2.2 Lesions that May Be Primary or Secondary

1) Alopecia refers to complete loss of hair whereas hypotrichosis is a partial loss of hair. Primary alopecia and hypotrichosis occur in conditions such as follicular dysplasia, follicular atrophy and other non-inflammatory diseases of the hair follicle. Secondary alopecia and hypotrichosis occur in pruritic skin conditions such as atopic dermatitis, cutaneous adverse food reaction, and ectoparasitic infestations. In secondary hypotrichosis and alopecia the hair loss is traumatically-induced and therefore the hairs will be broken.

2) A scale is a loose plate or fragment of stratum corneum. Scale is a primary lesion in primary keratinization defects such as ichthyosis. It is a secondary lesion in staphylococcal folliculitis.

3) A follicular cast is an accumulation of keratin and follicular material that adheres to hair shafts extending above the surface of the follicular ostia. Follicular casts are a primary lesion in certain keratinization defects such as sebaceous adenitis and a secondary lesion is canine demodecosis.

4) A comedo is a dilated hair follicle filled with cornified cells and sebaceous material. Comedones are a primary lesion in Schnauzer comedo syndrome. It is a secondary lesion in inflamed skin disease such as demodecosis

5) Pigmentary abnormalities are changes in skin color due to a variety of pigments or lack of pigment such as melanin. The most common pigmentary abnormalities are hyperpigmentation and hypopigmentation. Hyperpigmentation refers to increased melanin within the epidermis and often in dermal melanophages. It is often secondary in chronic inflammatory conditions and endocrinopathies but may be primary in neoplastic processes such as melanoma. Hypopigmentation refers to decreased melanin within the epidermis. It may be primary in disorders such as vitiligo and secondary in inflammatory, immune-mediated conditions of the basement membrane zone such as discoid lupus erythematosus.

4.2.3 Secondary Skin Lesions

1) An epidermal collarette is a special type of scale arranged in a circular rim of loose keratin flakes or peeling keratin. It is usually arranged around a central area of erythema or hyperpigmentation. Epidermal collarettes are most commonly due to a ruptured papule or pustule associated with staphylococcal folliculitis. They can also be seen in superficial pemphigus and other papular/pustular conditions.

2) Crust should be distinguished from scale on external examination. A crust is an accumulation of dried exudate, serum, pus, blood, cells, or keratin adherent to the skin surface.

3) A scar is an area of fibrous tissue that has replaced damaged dermis or subcutaneous tissue.

4) An excoriation is an erosion or ulcer caused by scratching, biting, or rubbing.

5) An erosion is a shallow epidermal defect that does not penetrate the basal laminar zone. An ulcer is a break in continuity of epidermis

with exposure of the underlying dermis. Distinguishing erosions and ulcerations can be difficult on gross examination.

6) A fissure is a linear cleft into the epidermis or through the epidermis into the dermis. A fissure may be single or multiple, curved, branching, or straight.

7) Lichenification is thickening and hardening of skin characterized by exaggeration of superficial skin markings. It is often associated with hyperpigmention. Hyperkeratosis is increased thickness of the stratum corneum.

8) A callus is a thickened, rough, hyperkeratotic, alopecic, often lichenified plaque.

4.3 Organ Examination, Sectioning, and Fixation

Carefully examine the skin of the entire carcass for lesions including mucocutaneous junctions, external ear canals, paw pads, nasal planum, claw beds, and the entire haired skin surface. If one or more claws/claw beds are abnormal, the digits should be collected for histopathologic examination.

In densely haired animals, carefully examine down to the skin. The carcass can be clipped for better exposure of the skin and in cases when trauma is suspected, reflecting the skin from the entire carcass allows for identification of areas of hemorrhage and bruising in the skin and subcutis.

4.3.1 Cytology

If there is only one or very few skin lesions, it is probably best to collect these lesions for histopathology. However, if there are numerous and widespread skin lesions, cytology can be a very helpful diagnostic tool. Touch impressions are easily made from lesions that are moist or greasy. Touch impression can also be made from underneath crusts, from fluid that is expressed from a lesion and from gently opening the surface of papules, pustules and vesicles. If a larger lesion has a draining tract, the surface should be cleaned and the lesion should be squeezed. The microscope slide is pressed directly against the site to be examined. Cytology from more solid nodular lesions can be taken with fine needle aspiration. Once the collected materials are allowed to dry on the slide, the slide can be stained with Diff-Quik®.

4.3.2 Skin Scrapes

In cases where mites are suspected, multiple skin scrapes from suspect lesions can be helpful in making a diagnosis. These are usually areas of hypotrichosis, alopecia, scale, or crust. First dip the scalpel blade in mineral oil and place a drop of oil on the microscope slide. The skin is scraped with a scalpel blade held at a 45–90° angle to the surface. Collected material is then gently wiped onto the surface of the microscope slide.

4.3.3 Hair Examination (Trichogram)

Plucking hairs from the skin and examining them under a microscope is called trichography. This can be a very useful tool in determining if hair loss is due to trauma (broken hairs) versus infectious causes such as dermatophytosis versus hereditary abnormalities of the hair shaft/follicle such as follicular dysplasia or color dilution alopecia versus other hair shaft/cycling abnormalities that would be difficult to diagnose with histopathology such as trichorrhexis nodosa, anagen defluxion, or telogen defluxion.

4.3.4 Examination of the External Ear Canal

Postmortem examination of the external ear canal can be performed with an otoscope. Any exudate can be collected with a clean swab and rolled onto a microscope slide for cytologic examination. If mites are suspected, material can be collected with a swab and placed on a microscope slide with a drop of mineral oil and a cover slip for cytologic examination. Tissue should be sampled for histopathologic examination if any masses are detected.

4.3.5 Sampling the Skin

Never closely shave or scrub the surface of skin that is being submitted for histopathology. This could remove important diagnostic information such as scales and crusts. Because the hair can dull the scalpel blade or punch biopsy instrument, it can be advantageous to trim hair with scissors or clippers (#40 blade) prior to procuring the samples. Trim above areas where there is abundant scaling and crusting.

Lesions should be obtained with a new 6 mm or greater diameter punch biopsy instrument or a new sharp scalpel blade. These instruments can be used multiple times in the same animal but do not use on multiple animals as they will dull easily after several uses and a dull blade or punch biopsy instrument with produce crushed samples.

To use a punch biopsy instrument, hold the instrument with one hand at right angles to the surface of the skin and place over the selected lesion. The surrounding skin should be held taut with the opposite hand. Apply firm continuous pressure and rotate the punch instrument in one direction until the instrument pops into the subcutis. Gently grasp the base of the sample with forceps. Cut the subcutaneous attachments with a scalpel blade or scissors.

To take an elliptical tissue sample, using a scalpel blade make an elliptical incision with one narrow end located within lesional tissue and the opposite narrow end located within normal tissue. Do not grasp the lesional end of the sample with tissue forceps as this leads to crush artifact. Crush artifact can greatly hinder the histologic evaluation.

Punch biopsy instruments should only be used if the entire lesion fits entirely within the diameter of the cutting surface of the punch instrument or for diffuse lesions in which large areas of the lesional skin have a similar appearance. For example, an entire pustule, diffuse area of erythema, or diffuse area of lichenification (Fig. 4.1).

For most lesions, especially primary lesions (papules, pustules, plaques, nodules, bullae, vesicles, cysts, wheals) the entire lesion should be collected *en bloc*. Elliptical and wedge biopsies should be used for larger lesions (nodules, neoplasms), and/or deep (panniculitis) and/or very fragile (big pustules, bullae, vesicles) lesions.

Placing the biopsy sample on a piece of tongue depressor or cardboard to minimize curling during fixation is optimal for thin biopsy specimens (not necessary for full thickness punch biopsies). Allow tissue to dry on the tongue depressor for 30–60 seconds before placing in formalin. Never attach the tissue to the tongue depressor or cardboard with needles or sutures, this will cause significant artifact.

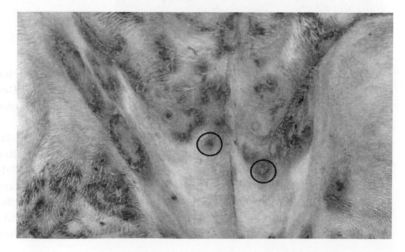

Figure 4.1 Multifocal to coalescing erythematous papules, pustules and epidermal collarettes on the ventral abdomen of a dog. A 6 mm punch biopsy instrument can fit over the entire papule.

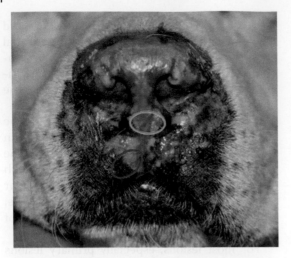

Figure 4.2 Ulcerative and depigmented macular and patch lesions on the nasal planum of a dog. Collect multiple elliptical samples at the margin of normal pigment and decreased pigment (red oval) and at the margin of ulcerated and non-ulcerated skin (green oval).

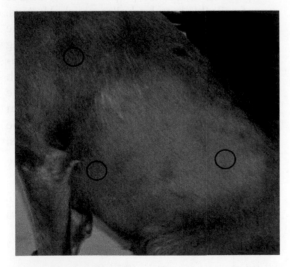

Figure 4.3 Hypotrichosis and alopecia on the trunk of a dog. Collect samples from areas that are most alopecic, partially hairless, and normal.

There are particular circumstances in which the margin of the lesion and normal skin is preferable and these include depigmenting lesions and ulcerative lesions. These types of lesions should be collected with a scalpel blade in an ellipse or wedge. For depigmenting lesions, collect gray areas or the margin between pigment and non-pigment (Fig. 4.2). For ulcerative lesions, collect the sample on the margin of intact skin extending into the ulcer (Fig. 4.2).

In cases where a significant proportion of the lesions are hypotrichosis and/or alopecia, collect samples from areas that are most alopecic, partially hairless and normal and label separately (Fig. 4.3).

4.4 Common Artifacts and Postmortem Changes

The skin usually holds up well in the immediate postmortem interval.

1) As in other organs, the dependent areas of the skin will often appear red due to gravitational settling of blood.
2) Hemoglobin imbibition can cause a diffuse red discoloration of the skin, particularly in animals that are frozen and thawed.
3) The skin of the abdomen may turn green secondary to bile imbibition and/or bacterial products from the adjacent intestine.

With prolonged postmortem intervals, the skin changes are more pronounced.

1) Skin sloughing and easy epilation of hair will be apparent in a carcass after 4–5 days.

Bibliography

Bettenay, SV, Hargis, AM. 2006. *Practical Veterinary Dermatopathology for the Small Animal Clinician*. Jackson, WY: Teton NewMedia.

Campbell, KL. 2004. *Small Animal Dermatology Secrets*. Paris: Elsevier.

Mauldin EA, Peters-Kennedy J. 2015. Integumentary system. In: *Jubb, Kennedy, and Palmer's Pathology of Domestic Animals, Volume 1*, 6th edn, pp. 509–736. New York: Saunders Elsevier.

Maxie, MG. 2015. Introduction to the diagnostic process. In: *Jubb, Kennedy, and Palmer's Pathology of Domestic Animals, Volume* 1, 6th edn, pp. 2–15. New York: Saunders Elsevier.

Miller WH. 2013. *Muller and Kirk's Small Animal Dermatology*, 7th edn. New York: Saunders Elsevier.

Presnell SE. *Postmortem changes*. [Available online] at: http://emedicine.medscape.com/article/1680032-overview#a5 (accessed August 8, 2016).

Wilcox BP, Njaa BL. 2015. Special senses. In: *Jubb, Kennedy, and Palmer's Pathology of Domestic Animals, Volume* 1, 6th edn, pp. 407–508. New York: Saunders Elsevier.

5

The Musculoskeletal System

5.1 Anatomy Review

In an average dog or cat, the musculoskeletal system consists of approximately 319 bones, over 300 joints, and more than 600 named skeletal muscles. The musculoskeletal system has a wide variety of functions including protection, movement, mineral storage, heat generation, and ventilation of the lungs. Necropsy examination of the musculoskeletal system is typically limited to external examination, rough assessment of bone strength, collection of representative sections of bone and muscle, and examination of multiple joints, unless the history or clinical signs warrant a more in-depth evaluation.

5.1.1 Bones and Joints

The bones are grouped into the axial skeleton (skull, vertebrae, scapulae, sternum, ribs, and pelvis), and the appendicular skeleton (limbs). Bones can also be classified as long bones, short bones, flat bones, and irregular bones. This classification is important in understanding development of the skeletal system (flat bones undergo intramembranous ossification and the other types undergo endochondral ossification) and because susceptibility to some disease processes varies among the types of bones.

The skull (Fig. 5.1) consists of 14 paired and 7 unpaired bones, with more than 40 foramina that allow for the passage of vessels and nerves. These bones can be divided into the calvaria, or skull cap (dorsal parts of the frontal, occipital, and parietal), the base of the skull (ventral parts of the frontal, parietal, and occipital; sphenoid, temporal, and ethmoid) and facial bones (maxilla, mandible, nasal, lacrimal, palatine, incisive, pterygoid, vomer, zygomatic, and nasal conchae). The only synovial joints in the head are the temporomandibular joints and the atlanto-occipital joint. Other joints are synarthroses or sutures, which may be open at birth, but typically close by 6 weeks of age or, less commonly, by 6 months of age. Initially, these joints are fused by fibrous connective tissue, but they may become ossified in older animals.

The vertebral column consists of 7 cervical, 13 thoracic, 7 lumbar, 3 fused sacral, and a variable number (20–23) of coccygeal or caudal vertebrae. Vertebrae are classified as irregular bones and are formed through endochondral ossification. The parts of a typical vertebra are labeled in Fig. 5.2. The first cervical vertebra, or the atlas, articulates with the occipital condyles of the skull (Fig. 5.3). Other vertebrae articulate with their cranial and caudal neighbors via facets. The transverse processes of the thoracic vertebrae articulate with the heads of the ribs. Ribs are flat bones, composed of a dorsal ossified part and a ventral cartilaginous part. The ribs also articulate with the eight sternebrae, which are connected by intersternebral cartilages. The manubrium is the first sternebra and the xiphoid process is the last sternebra.

The hyoid apparatus (stylohyoid, epihyoid, ceratohyoid, basihyoid, and thyrohyoid; Fig. 5.4)

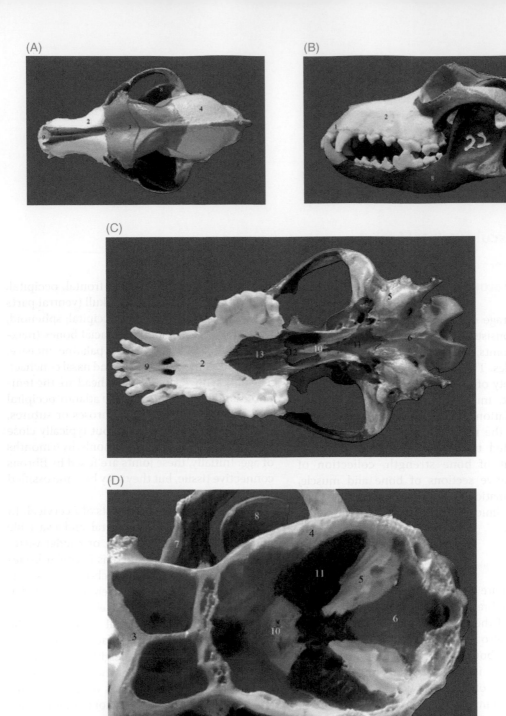

Figure 5.1 Dorsal (A), lateral (B), and ventral (C) views of the intact canine skull, and a dorsal view inside of the calvaria (D). The bones of the skull are labeled as follows: 1. Nasal bone; 2. Maxilla; 3. Frontal bone; 4. Parietal bone; 5. Temporal bone; 6. Occipital bone; 7. Zygomatic bone; 8. Mandible; 9. Incisive bone; 10. Presphenoid bone; 11. Basisphenoid bone; 12. Vomer; 12. Palatine bone.

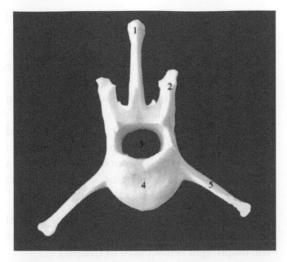

Figure 5.2 Parts of a canine lumbar vertebra: 1. Spinous process; 2. Articular process; 3. Vertebral foramen; 4. Body; 5. Transverse process.

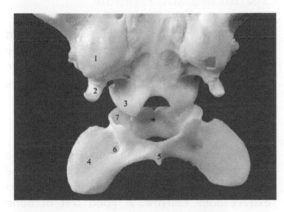

Figure 5.3 Parts of the atlanto-occipital joint: 1. Tympanic bulla; 2. Jugular process; 3. Occipital condyle; 4. Transverse process (wing) of the atlas; 5. Ventral tubercle of the atlas; 6. Transverse foramen of the atlas; and 7. Cranial articular fossa.

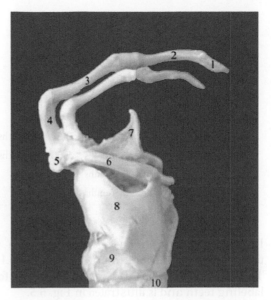

Figure 5.4 Bones of the hyoid apparatus and laryngeal cartilages. Lateral view. 1. Tympanohyoid; 2. Stylohyoid; 3. Epihyoid, 4. Ceratohyoid; 5. Baslhyoid; 6. Thyrohyoid; 7. Epiglottis; 8. Thyroid cartilage; 9. Cricoid cartilage; and 10. Trachea.

and the ossicles of the inner ear (incus, malleus, and stapes) are also part of the axial skeleton.

The bones of the forelimb include the scapula, humerus, radius, ulna, carpal bones (radial, ulnar, accessory, first, second, third, and fourth), metacarpal bones, and phalanges (proximal, middle, and distal). Cats and dogs have a rudimentary clavicle. The hindlimb bones are the pelvic bones (ischium, ilium, and pubis), femur, patella, tibia, fibula, tarsal bones (talus, calcaneus, central, first, second, third, and fourth), metatarsal bones, and phalanges (proximal, middle, and distal).

5.1.2 Teeth

Cat and dog teeth are brachydont, or low crowned, and consist of three parts: crown (above the gingiva), neck (at the gingival margin), and root (embedded in the alveolar bone). The pulp cavity, which houses the nerves and blood vessels, is encased in a layer of bone-like dentin. The crown of the tooth is covered with enamel and the root is covered with cementum. The surfaces of a tooth are referred to as mesial (toward the center of the arcade), distal (away from the center of the arcade), labial (facing the lip), lingual (facing the tongue), and occlusal (surface that opposes the opposite tooth when the jaws are closed). The dental formula of a dog is i3/3 c1/1 p3/3 for deciduous teeth and I3/3 C1/1 P4/4 M2/3 for permanent teeth. For cats, the formula is i3/3 c1/1 p3/2 and I3/3 C1/1

Table 5.1 Age of teeth eruption in dogs and cats.

	Dog	Cat
Deciduous incisors	4–6 weeks	3–4 weeks
Deciduous canines	5–6 weeks	3–4 weeks
Deciduous premolars	6 weeks	6 weeks
Permanent incisors	3–5 months	3.5–5.5 months
Permanent canines	4–6 months	5.5–6.5 months
Permanent premolars	4–5 months	4.5 months
Permanent molars	5–7 months	5–6 months

P3/2 M1/1. The pattern of tooth eruption is useful in estimating an animal's age (Table 5.1). The triadont system is the preferred method for labeling teeth and is illustrated in Fig. 5.5.

5.1.3 Skeletal Muscle

Skeletal muscle comprises approximately half of the body mass of an animal. For the most part, all skeletal muscles have similar structure: They are fusiform or flattened bands composed of bundles of myofibers (muscle cells) that are filled with myofibrils composed of overlapping myofilaments. Each of these layers is invested in a sheath of connective tissue. Skeletal muscles attach, via tendons, to one fixed and one mobile surface (usually bone, but also cartilage or other tissue types). Despite the similarity in structure and function, susceptibility to disease processes can vary significantly among muscle groups, depending on a variety of factors: location (axial vs appendicular), function (gravity vs antigravity), size (large vs small), and predominant fiber type (I, IIA, IIB in cats or I, IIA, IIX in dogs).

The skeletal muscles that are cut during the standard necropsy procedure include:

Superficial and deep pectorals – cut when reflecting the right forelimb
Hindlimb adductors (gracilis, pectineus, adductor, and external obturator) – cut when reflecting the hind limb
Abdominal muscles (rectus abdominus, transversus abdominus, internal, and external oblique – cut when opening the abdominal cavity (Fig. 5.6)
Diaphragm, intercostal muscles, trapezius, latissimus dorsi – cut when opening the thorax
Digastric and stylohyoid muscles – cut when extracting the tongue from the oral cavity
Strap muscles of the neck (sternohyoid and omohyoid), ventral neck muscles (longus colli and longus capitis), dorsal neck muscles (splenius, obliquus capitis caudalis) – cut when taking off the head.

A skeletal muscle which deserves special consideration is the diaphragm. The anatomy of the diaphragm is discussed in Chapter 7.

5.2 *In Situ* Evaluation, Sectioning, and Fixation

Examination of the musculoskeletal system begins with the external exam. Observe the body for evidence of asymmetry, atrophy, deformity, and palpate for swelling, crepitus, and abnormal motility.

5.2.1 Bones

Bone strength and mineralization can be roughly assessed as the ribs are cut to open the thoracic cavity and when the femur is opened to extract bone marrow. A good test of bone strength in an adult animal is to manually attempt to break a rib from the section of thoracic wall that was removed to access the thoracic cavity (see Fig. 3.24). The rib should snap when a moderate amount of force is applied. If the rib breaks with minimal force or bends with no distinct snap, further investigation of underlying bone disease is warranted and a sample of bone should be included in the formalin-fixed tissue submitted for histopathology. The skeleton is more flexible in puppies and kittens, so the ribs often bend rather than snapping. In young animals, the costochondral junction can be assessed by shaving off the cranial or caudal edge of a rib (Fig. 5.7).

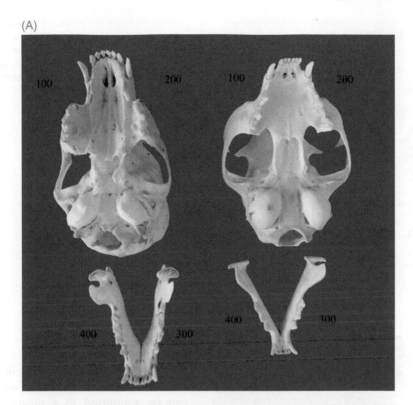

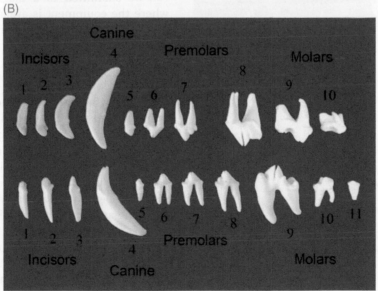

Figure 5.5 Canine and feline dental arcades are labeled using the triadan system in (A). (B) shows half of the canine complement of adult teeth. The arcades are designated as 100s (right maxillary), 200s (left maxillary), 300s (left mandibular), and 400s (right mandibular). In dogs, the incisors are designated 1–3, the canines are 4, premolars are 5–8, and molars are 9–10 (maxillary) and 9–11 (mandibular). In cats, the incisors and canines are the same, but the mandibular premolars are 7–8, the maxillary premolars are 6–8, and the single molars are designated 9.

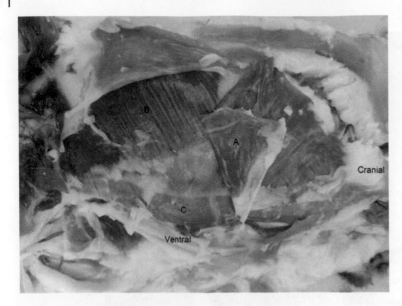

Figure 5.6 The layers of body wall muscles that are cut when the abdomen is opened. A. External oblique (partially reflected); B. Internal oblique; and C. Rectus abdominus.

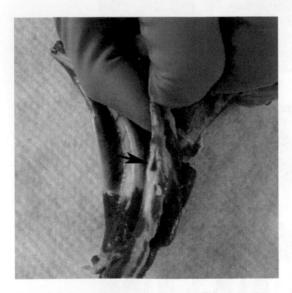

Figure 5.7 In young animals, shaving off the cranial edge of a rib at the costrochondral junction allows for assessment for changes compatible with rickets. In old dogs, the cartilage of the costochondral junction often undergoes dystrophic mineralization, a change of no significance.

Any lesions involving the bone, either detected on the necropsy examination or with pre- or postmortem imaging, should be thoroughly investigated, first by removing the skin from the affected area and then by dissecting the surrounding soft tissue. An oscillating saw can be used to take a sample of a bony lesion for formalin fixation. Alternatively, an entire fresh limb can be submitted to a diagnostic laboratory where the equipment is available to take samples and remove the soft tissue from the bone for further evaluation.

5.2.2 Joints, Tendons, and Ligaments

Four joints (the right coxofemoral, stifle, glenohumoral, and the atlanto-occipital) are opened as part of the standard necropsy procedure. At least one additional joint should be opened in an adult animal and three additional joints in a young animal. The choice of joints to open should depend on the history and signalment. In young animals, the tarsal (hock) joints are a good choice because these are large joints and common sites of fibrinous arthritis in a septic animal. In geriatric animals, degenerative changes are most commonly seen in the coxofemoral, femorotibial, humeroradial, and glenohumoral joints, so these should be opened bilaterally. Opening joints requires cutting through the surrounding skin, muscle, tendons, and fascia, incising the joint capsule and cutting

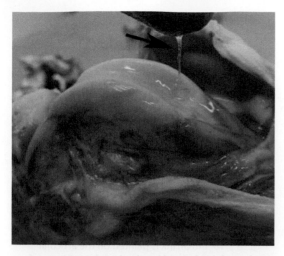

Figure 5.8 Synovial fluid should be clear, colorless to light yellow, and viscous enough to be stretched several centimeters with a gloved finger. Changes in the color or consistency may be secondary to inflammation.

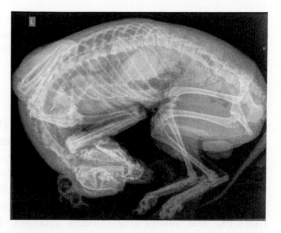

Figure 5.9 A postmortem, whole body radiograph of a dog can be used to assess the bones and look for metal projectiles.

the ligaments. Palpate the joint through the range of motion to find the right place to cut. Restrictions in the range of motion or crepitus should be assessed at this time. The joint should be opened so that the entire articular surface is exposed for evaluation. Normal synovial fluid is clear, colorless to straw colored, and has sufficient viscosity to be stretched at least several centimeters between two gloved fingers (Fig. 5.8). Loss of viscosity is associated with inflammation. Another indication of inflammation is aggregates of friable tan material (fibrin) within the joint. The articular cartilage should be white, smooth, and shiny. Exposure of subchondral bone on an articular surface can be observed as a color change and area of depression, or demonstrated by tapping an instrument (dull side of the knife blade or scalpel handle) on the surface: tapping against cartilage gives a dull sound, while exposed bone produces more of a sharp sound.

5.2.3 Skeletal Muscle

The skeletal muscle is evaluated in the external examination, as the carcass is opened, and as joints are opened. A section of biceps femoris

muscle is collected, along with sciatic nerve and skin, in a routine necropsy (See Fig. 3.17). Additional samples should be collected as is appropriate, based on the history and necropsy findings. Samples of muscle, like skin and nerve, will curl up during fixation unless attached to a flat surface. A disposable muscle biopsy clamp provides excellent orientation. Alternatively, a wooden tongue depressor or piece of cardboard can be used to flatten out these sections. The tissues should be allowed to dry for a minute or two before being placed in formalin. Some pathologists staple muscle samples to cardboard to ensure that the sample remains attached during fixation. The tongue depressor or cardboard can easily be labeled with the location of the muscle using a number 2 pencil.

5.3 Special Techniques

5.3.1 Postmortem Imaging

Often skeletal lesions are not found at necropsy unless the prosector knows where to look. If antemortem films are not available, dead animals are very cooperative, although not necessarily very flexible, imaging patients (Fig. 5.9).

A whole body radiograph can be used to guide a careful dissection of areas of interest and allow appropriate sections to be collected for histopathology.

5.3.2 Cleaning Bones

Bony lesions can often be best assessed when all of the soft tissue is removed. Soft tissue removal can be achieved by boiling the sample or, where available, allowing a colony of dermestid beetles to clean soft tissues from the bones. These techniques are helpful in assessing fractures, malformations, and severe degenerative changes. If histopathology is also desired, a section from the edge of the lesion can be collected in formalin prior to cleaning the bones. Remove as much soft tissue as possible first. Next, soak them in hot water (85 °C/185 °F) with dish detergent, being sure to check every few hours as excess cooking can degrade the bone matrix. If degreasing is necessary, soak the bones in either acetone or concentrated Dawn dish detergent (it can be discharged into a sanitary sewer drain). A soak in 7–15% hydrogen peroxide will brighten the bones but commercial 3% hydrogen peroxide available from a retail pharmacy will also work.

5.3.3 India Ink Evaluation of Articular Cartilage

India ink, when painted onto articular surfaces, will adhere to areas of fissures, and allow visualization and quantification of cartilage damage. The ink does not adhere to exposed subchondral bone. A 20% solution of ink in a phosphate buffered saline is recommended. This solution is painted on the cartilage and left for 15 seconds (Fig. 5.10) before blotting the excess off with a moist cotton swab.

5.3.4 Examining the Intervertebral Discs

Examination of the intervertebral discs usually follows removal of the spinal cord (see Chapter 11 for instructions). Once the cord is removed, the vertebral canal can be examined

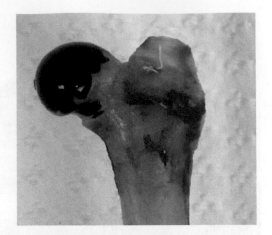

Figure 5.10 Indian ink is painted on the articular surface of this femoral head to look for evidence of cartilage damage. The ink is wiped off with saline.

for evidence of disc protrusion or rupture. Bone cutting forceps or an oscillating saw can be used to longitudinally section the vertebral column (Fig. 5.11) and to collect a sample for histopathology.

5.3.5 Submitting Muscle for Additional Tests

Testing for muscular dystrophies, congenital myopathies, acetylcholine receptor antibodies, and inborn errors of metabolism requires special handling of samples. Most of this testing is performed at the Comparative Neuromuscular Laboratory at the University of California, San Diego (http://vetneuromuscular.ucsd.edu/). Consultation with the laboratory website or personnel is recommended if this type of testing is desired.

5.4 Common Artifacts and Postmortem Changes

The cells of bone and muscle tissues have relatively low numbers of lysosomes and, therefore, these tissues are somewhat resistant to postmortem decomposition; however, the prosector

Figure 5.11 Once the spinal cord is removed, the vertebral canal can be sectioned with an oscillating saw to examine the vertebral canal and intervertebral discs.

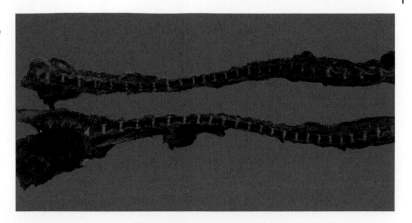

should be aware of the following postmortem changes:

1) The color of skeletal muscle can vary significantly (from dark red to light grey) depending on the degree of autolysis.
2) Postmortem fractures can result from handling of the carcass, and should be distinguished from antemortem fractures by the absence of swelling, hemorrhage, and local tissue reaction.
3) The articular cartilage may have discontinuities in areas away from the articular surface (synovial fossae), which should not be interpreted as erosions.
4) Rigor mortis is the postmortem contraction of skeletal muscle secondary to release of calcium from intracellular stores. The contractions usually begin several hours after death, starting at the jaw and progressing to the axial and limb muscles, and peak in 24–48 h before starting to dissipate.

Resolution of rigor mortis proceeds in the same order as it formed. The rate and degree of rigor mortis depend on temperature, muscle glycogen stores, pH, total muscle mass, and amount of muscle activity prior to death.

Bibliography

Boyd, JS. 2001. *Color Atlas of Clinical Anatomy of the Dog and Cat*, 2nd edn. London: Mosby, International.

Dyce DM, Sack WO, Wensing, CJG. 1996. *Textbook of Veterinary Anatomy*, 2nd edn, Ch. 2, 12, 16, and 17. Philadelphia, PA: W.B. Saunders Company.

Schmitz N, Laverty S, Kraus VB, Aigner, T. 2010. Basic methods in histopathology of joint tissues. *Osteoarthritis and Cartilage* 18(Supplement 3): S113–116.

6

The Cardiovascular System

6.1 Anatomy Review

The cardiovascular system consists of the heart, arteries, veins, and connecting vascular beds. The heart is an ovoid (in the dog) to valentine (in the cat), asymmetric muscular dual pump structure. The right heart provides for the functional pulmonary circulation while the left side of the heart supplies the systemic circulation; the relative thickness of the ventricular walls reflects the differences in work load. The external anatomy of the heart is distinguished by two atrial appendages/auricles and an array of vascular structures at the heart base. The left ventricle forms the apex of the heart with the right ventricle spiraling across the ventral surface. Prominent coronary vessels (arteries and veins) embedded in epicardial fat in the coronary sulcus demarcate the approximate positions of the different cardiac chambers (atria and ventricles). The chambers of atria and ventricles are separated by atrioventricular (AV) valves that are supported by chordae tendineae to prevent valve eversion during systole. The pulmonic and aortic valves are semilunar and lack chordae.

6.1.1 Right Heart

The right heart receives systemic venous return from the cranial and caudal venae cavae; on the dorsal aspect, the junction of the venae cavae with the right atrium is marked by a groove (the sulcus terminalis). Blood is diverted from the cava into the right atrium due to a crest of tissue (intervenous tubercle). The fossa ovalis, a remnant of the foramen ovale, forms an oval shaped depression within the dorsal aspect of the interatrial septum. This structure will be probe patent, but functionally closed *in situ*, until several weeks after birth. The right atrial appendage is roughly triangular with an undulating inner muscular surface (pectinate muscles). The coronary sinus, receiving blood from the coronary veins, is present in the dorsal aspect of the right atrium at the atrioventricular junction proximal to the septal leaflet of the tricuspid valve. The tricuspid/right atrioventricular valve separates the right atrium and ventricle. In dogs, septal (dorsal) and parietal (ventral) leaflets can be fused thus appearing as the valve only has two cusps. In some cases, small secondary cusps are located at the extremities of these two large cusps. The free edges of valve leaflets are supported by fibrous chordae tendineae extending to broad trabecular papillary muscles or to the septum. In the dog, there are usually three papillary muscles; however, the arrangement of the papillary muscles is highly variable with bifed and occasionally trifed papillary muscles due to fusion of the bases, which has no clinical significance. The lumen of the right ventricle is crescent-shaped with a muscular strut, the trabecula septomarginalis (moderator band), passing through the lumen from the free wall to the interventricular septum and carrying the right bundle branch of the conduction system. The apical ventricular

Necropsy Guide for Dogs, Cats, and Small Mammals, First Edition. Edited by Sean P. McDonough and Teresa Southard.
© 2017 John Wiley & Sons, Inc. Published 2017 by John Wiley & Sons, Inc.
Companion Website: www.wiley.com/go/mcdonough/necropsy

lumen is lined by muscular bundles or trabeculae (trabeculae carneae). The pulmonary artery is rather prominently positioned on the ventral heart base to the left of the aorta; the gateway to the pulmonary circulation is the pulmonic semilunar valve, which has three cusps. The crista supraventricularis, an ultrasound landmark for the RV inflow and outflow tracts, is a muscular shelf along the septal curvature separating the right AV and pulmonic valves.

6.1.2 Left Heart

In the dog, the left atrium receives blood from the pulmonary circulation via a variable number of pulmonary veins while the cat has four pulmonary veins. The left atrial appendage has a similar triangular shape to the right. The mitral valve/left AV valve is composed of two leaflets: a larger, saddle shaped anterior/ventral (septal) leaflet and a smaller posterior/dorsal (parietal) leaflet. Both are attached via chordae to prominent anterior and posterior papillary

muscles (Fig. 6.1). The anterior leaflet is also connected to the aortic valve and contributes to the left ventricular outflow tract (Fig. 6.2, image 6). The interventricular (IV) septum separates the left and right ventricle but is functionally part of the left ventricle. The aorta emerges from the center of the heart. The ostia of coronary arteries are located in dilations of the proximal aorta (sinuses of Valsava) adjacent to the cusps of the aortic semilunar valve. It is expected to have two coronary and one non-coronary sinus of Valsalva. Nodular thickenings are present in the center of the free edge of the aortic semilunar valve leaflets (Nodules of Arantius), which may enhance valve coaptation.

6.1.3 Vessels: Great and Small

The vascular or circulatory system conducts blood from the heart (arterial system), systemically through the tissues, and then back to the heart (venous system); it encompasses the arteries, arterioles, capillaries, post-capillary venules,

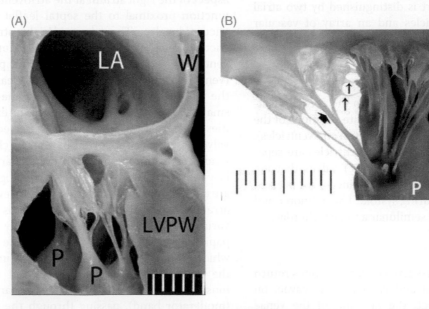

Figure 6.1 A. Sagittal section of normal canine mitral valve apparatus, left atrium, and left ventricle. The normal mitral valve annulus and orientation to associated structures, including the left atrium (LA), LA wall (W), and left ventricular posterior wall (LVPW). The normal mitral valve/left AV valve leaflets are thin and translucent.
B. Transilluminated normal canine mitral valve apparatus. The normal mitral valve/left AV valve leaflets are attached via first (small arrows) and second order (broad arrow) chordae tendineae to left ventricle papillary muscle (P). Figures reprinted from *Journal of Veterinary Cardiology*, 14/1, Philip R. Fox, Pathology of myxomatous mitral valve disease in the dog, Pages 103–126, Copyright (2012), with permission from Elsevier.

Figure 6.2 Flow of blood (inflow/outflow) dissection of the canine heart. 1. Ventral aspect of the heart. 2. Dorsal aspect of the heart with truncated pulmonary veins. 3. Dorsal aspect of the heart base emphasizing the orientation of great vessels: caudal vena cava (blue), aorta (red), pulmonary artery (green), and pulmonary veins (tan sketch overlay). 4. Dorsal aspect of the heart opened from the caudal vena cava to the tip of the right atrial appendage exposing the right atrial lumen and right AV valve. 5. Lateral aspect of the heart with the right ventricular free wall removed accentuating the crescent shape of the right ventricle lumen. 6. The left ventricular (LV) outflow tract of the heart with a portion of the LV removed.

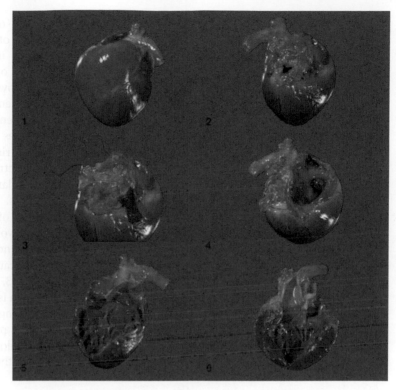

and veins. With few exceptions, the arterial system carries oxygenated blood (exceptions: pulmonary arteries, umbilical arteries) while veins carry deoxygenated blood (exceptions: pulmonary vein, umbilical vein). In general, blood vessels have a basic three-layered structure: the inner most tunica intima, which supports the endothelium, the tunica media composed of variable smooth muscle cells and connective tissue fibers, and the tunica adventitia that blends into adjacent connective tissue. The thickness or existence of individual layers depends on pressure within the vessel lumen.

The trilaminar architecture is most apparent in arteries. There are several types of arteries: elastic arteries, muscular arteries (which branch into successively smaller diameter), and the arterioles. The tunica media of elastic arteries contains amounts of elastin and collagen that allows for elastic recoil and the conduction of blood. Elastic arteries are the largest in the body and have already been mentioned during the discussion of

the heart: the pulmonary artery and the aorta. Muscular arteries are also known as distributing arteries with a tunica media that includes a more prominent spiraled layer of smooth muscle. Arterioles are the smallest arteries and give rise to microscopic, thin-walled capillaries where nutrient, waste, and gas exchange occurs.

Venules collect blood from capillary beds and merge to form successively larger veins that ultimately drain into the right atrium. Veins have valves which prevent back flow of blood in this low pressure system. On cross section, veins have a thinner wall to luminal diameter versus a companion artery.

In parallel, the lymphatic system begins as blind-ended lymphatics that recapture the excess of fluid lost into the interstitium around the tissue microcirculation. Like veins, lymphatics merge to form successively larger vessels with valves. The lymphatic system drains into lymph nodes before rejoining the venous system via the thoracic and tracheal ducts.

6.1.4 Contextual Cardiac Embryology and Congenital Heart Malformations

Few veterinarians fondly recall learning the embryology of the heart; however, a basic understanding of this process is important to appreciating normal cardiac anatomy and provides the conceptual framework for understanding congenital heart disease. The complexity of cardiac development allows the embryo to maintain constant blood flow to organs and the placenta while changing from a simple symmetric tube to a multi- chambered, dual pump structure with fully separated systemic and pulmonary pathways.

The transformation into the four-chambered heart involves looping of the simple cardiac tube followed by formation of a series of partial or complete septa; these are the atrio-ventricular (A-V), interventricular (IV), and interatrial (IA) septa within the heart and the spiral septum of the outflow tract (Fig. 6.3). The formation of intracardiac septa is accomplished by development of endocardial cushions, which are regions of specialized endothelial cells. Because the inflow and outflow tracks are tethered, the original cardiac tube rotates and loops as it grows. This brings the early ventricle caudal and ventral to the atrium, and sets up the realignment of the atrium so that the A-V canal overlies the middle of the common (bulbo) ventricle. Partial separation of the common ventricle is initiated but leaves an interventricular foramen to be closed later in cardiogenesis.

Separation of the single atrium into left and right atria involves the sequential formation of two membranous interatrial septa that grow cranially to caudally and do not fully close in utero (Fig. 6.3, left panels). This complexity of atrial division is an embryologic adaptation that allows shunting of oxygenated blood away from lungs as well providing a mechanism to block inter-atrial blood flow at birth. Due to the resistance of the pulmonary bed in the embryo,

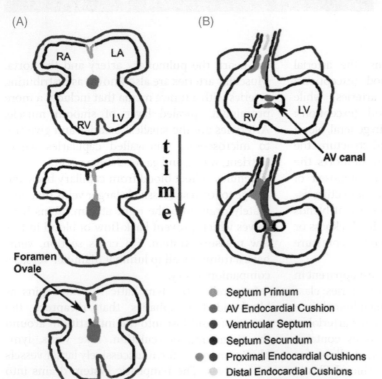

(A)   (B)

RA   LA

RV   LV

RV   LV

AV canal

Foramen Ovale

● Septum Primum
● AV Endocardial Cushion
● Ventricular Septum
● Septum Secundum
●● Proximal Endocardial Cushions
○ Distal Endocardial Cushions

Figure 6.3 Schematic of septation during cardiac development. Right atrium (RA), left atrium (LA), right ventricle (RV), and left ventricle (LV). A. Coronal section of the fetal heart demonstrating sequence of atrial and ventricular septation. B. Caudo-ventral oblique section demonstrating the endocardial cushions during the separation of the single outflow tract into the aorta and pulmonary artery and completion of ventricular septum. The perpendicular distal endocardial cushion is removed.

blood flows from right to the left through the interatrial foramina. At birth, with opening of the pulmonary capillary bed and cessation of placental blood flow, the pressure gradient reverses which pushes the septa together thereby blocking inter-atrial blood flow. These septa fuse after birth; however, a depression, the fossa ovalis, remains in the right atrium. Occasionally, the foramen ovale may remain probe patent but is functionally closed due to the difference in atrial pressures.

Blood flows through the embryonic outflow tract, the proximal bulbus cordis and truncus arteriosus, and then cranially through the aortic arches. Two perpendicularly oriented pairs of endocardial cushions within the outflow tract fuse in different planes creating a twisting membrane, the spiral septum (Fig. 6.3, left panels). Elongation of the proximal pair of these (bulbar) endocardial cushions also contributes to closure of the interventricular foramen. Closure of the interventricular foramen completes separation of the left and right ventricles and links them with systemic and pulmonary blood flow.

In addition to the foramen ovale, there is an extracardiac shunt in the fetus that diverts blood from the pulmonary vasculature until after parturition: the ductus arteriosus. The ductus is the dorsal part of the left sixth aortic arch, and serves to shunt blood from the pulmonary artery to the aorta. Its wall is composed of a combination of smooth muscle and elastic tissue (more aorta-like). In most species, the ductus closes within hours of birth; once constricted, it is the ligamentum arteriosum. Failure of this channel to close after birth results in a patent ductus arteriosus (PDA).

Heart development is spatiotemporally complex and requires a balance between intrinsic programming and hemodynamic pressures. Congenital heart malformations are usually due to incomplete or incorrect formation of endocardial cushions and septa. If any of the cushions develop incorrectly (i.e., incorrect position or time) left and right blood flows may not fully separate resulting in outflow tract problems. A striking clinical example is Tetralogy of Fallot, a suite of three primary and one secondary cardiac lesions. This abnormality results from off-centered development of the bulbar cushion contributing to the spiral septum which is shifted towards the right side of the developing heart. The result is a narrow opening into the pulmonary trunk (pulmonic stenosis, PS). The opening into the aortic root is correspondingly too large and expanded on the right side (dextro-aorta). The off-center cushions also fail to fuse with the interventricular septum, resulting in a septal defect. As the PS causes increased resistance to RV ejection of blood, right ventricular hypertrophy develops secondarily.

6.2   *In Situ* Evaluation and Removal

The *in situ* examination of the heart is accomplished after opening the thorax. The subcutis, abdominal, and thoracic cavities should be assessed for fluid with appropriate sampling (fluid analysis, cytology, bacterial culture, etc.). Once the thoracic cavity is opened and before any organs are removed, the heart in its pericardial sac, the lungs, great vessels, and mediastinal structures should be examined for their size and position. The heart occupies an asymmetric position with the apex of the heart pointed into the left hemithorax. The size of the heart relative to the thorax can be observed as a possible indicator of cardiac hypertrophy. The heart is enclosed in the pericardial sac, which is normally thin and translucent. Chronic pericardial sac disease results in fibrous thickening and increased vascularity. The venae cavae are present to the right of dorsal midline, while the aorta originates from the center of the heart base and then arches to the left and dorsally to a dorsal midline position ventral to the vertebral bodies. While still *in situ*, a small window can be cut in the pericardial sac allowing careful examination for fluid, clotted blood, or other pericardial contents (including other organs!).

The approximate amount of fluid should be noted with appropriate sampling of pericardial content (fluid analysis, cytology, bacterial culture, etc.) before organ removal. The serous layer of the parietal pericardium (i.e., the inner surface) must be inspected carefully for roughening or discoloration that may indicate pericarditis, uremic mineralization, or even pericardial sac mesothelioma. The incision can then be extended to allow complete eversion of the heart and an opportunity to examine the pulmonary veins returning to the left atrium.

The caudal vena cava, aorta and esophagus should be cut rostral to the diaphragm as the heart is then removed as part of the pluck (see Chapter 2: Necropsy Basics) leaving the aorta and other great vessels attached. The vascular connections between the heart and lungs are examined closely before removal of the heart from the pluck. When congenital heart disease is suspected, the heart should be left attached to the lungs which provides important landmarks during cardiac dissection (see congenital defect section). In addition, if pulmonary vascular disease is suspected (i.e., heartworm disease), preserving the pulmonary artery and vein connections facilitates examination of the pulmonary vasculature. If these connections are not considered necessary for cardiac dissection, the heart can be removed by transecting the aorta and pulmonary artery at the heart base and leaving approximately 5 cm of the vessels attached. The apex of the heart is then lifted to reveal and allow transection of the right and left pulmonary veins as they enter the dorsal ventral aspect of the left atrium.

Due to the collapsible nature of vessels and shifting of organs, it is best to examine the major blood supply of a particular organ *in situ* and sample prior to removal if disease is suspected. The abdominal aorta is best observed *in situ*. It can be observed ventral to the vertebral bodies with minimal blunt dissection through the associated adipose tissue and can be opened along its length.

6.3 Organ Examination, Sectioning, and Fixation

The epicardial surface of the heart normally has fat, particularly in the epicardial sulci surrounding the coronary vessels. The amount of fat may be dramatic in obese animals. The heart should be examined externally to identify the ventricles and atria, and assess color, texture, and consistency. Fibrovascular epicardial proliferations often correspond to chronic heart dilation.

Detailed measurements to determine the presence of hypertrophy or dilation are available for the dog; however, at minimum, the total body weight/heart weight should be determined if cardiac disease is suspected. The heart should be weighed after removal of clotted blood. In normal adult dogs, the heart should be approximately 0.76% of the body weight (0.58–0.94%). In the young, the heart usually represents a larger proportion of body weight. In the cat the heart should represent 0.47% of lean body mass. While crude, a cut off heart weight of 20 g is used as an indicator of cardiac hypertrophy in the cat.

An understanding of cardiac anatomy is a key component to approaching examination of the heart. There are several cardiac dissection methods (including flow of blood, tomographic, bread-loafing techniques) that can be considered on the basis of the case signalment, history, and the results of antemortem diagnostics including imaging. Each method has advantages and disadvantages. The tools required for the dissection of the heart are relatively simple and include scissors, knife, scalpel, and flush (saline is ideal but water will work, although the color of the heart will fade).

When a congenital heart defect is suspected it is extremely helpful to leave the heart attached to the lungs and use a dissection approach that follows the flow of blood (inflow/outflow dissection). Severe cardiac abnormalities can cause distortion of expected cardiac landmarks but in most cases connection of the pulmonary vasculature and aorta, or lack thereof, may provide orientation. This method also preserves the

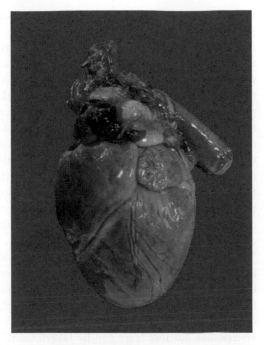

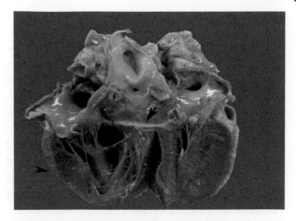

Figure 6.5 The left ventricular (LV) outflow tract of the heart from a Staffordshire Bull Terrier mix puppy with multiple congenital heart abnormalities. The LV outflow tract should be examined closely for stenosis or other areas of fibrosis. A complete subvalvular band of white connective tissue is prominent in the outflow tract. Compensatory left ventricular hyperplasia was prominent but difficult to appreciate as the LV is sectioned through the anterior papillary muscle (arrow).

Figure 6.4 The ventral aspect of the heart from a golden retriever dog with left auricular hemangiosarcoma. During a cardiac necropsy, the tip of the atrial appendage should be examined closely for neoplasia, particularly in cases with hemopericardium.

landmarks of the conduction system. The entry of the venae cavae should be identified on the dorsal aspect of the heart (Fig. 6.2, images 2 and 3). The right atrium can then be opened beginning at the caudal vena cava and continuing to the tip of the right atrial appendage, preserving the junction of the cranial vena cava and right atrium and the landmarks for the sinoatrial node (Fig. 6.2, image 4). The tip of the atrial appendage should be examined closely for neoplasia (i.e., hemangiosarcoma), particularly in cases with hemopericardium (Fig. 6.4). After examination of the right atrioventricular valve to exclude disease (dysplasia, endocardiosis, vegetations, etc.), the right ventricle is opened along the dorsal aspect of the free wall where it joins the septum and continued to the apex of the right ventricle (Fig. 6.2, image 5). This cut is continued along the ventral aspect of the heart and into the pulmonary trunk following the

crescent shape of the right ventricular lumen. The right ventricular outflow tract should be examined for stenotic bands. As the cut extends into the pulmonary artery, it should be shifted toward the left/lateral side to facilitate assessment of the ductus arteriosus.

The left atrium is opened by cutting along the lateral margin. After inspection of the mitral valve to exclude disease, this cut is extended to the apex of the left ventricle between the papillary muscles. The left atrioventricular valve may be variably distorted by smooth nodular to coalescing areas (myxomatous mitral valve disease/endocardiosis) particularly in dogs, which is clinically significant if associated with dilation/valvular regurgitation. To examine the left ventricular outflow tract, aortic valve, and aorta incise the anterior leaflet of the left AV valve (Fig. 6.2, image 6). The left ventricular outflow tract should be examined closely for stenosis or other areas of fibrosis (Fig. 6.5). The origin of the coronary arteries should be observed within the corresponding sinus with the opening (ostia) at or below the sinotubular junction. Although coronary artery disease is relatively rare in veterinary species, the coronary arteries should be opened with a small pair of scissors.

As the flow of blood technique does not allow for visualization of much of the myocardium, short-axis sectioning/bread loaf technique is most appropriate for suspected infiltrative disease (lymphoma, myocarditis, myocardial fibrosis, amyloidosis, etc.) and/or cardiomyopathy. With the ventral aspect of the heart placed down on the cutting surface, a series of 1–2 cm thick short axis sections are made through the ventricles from apex towards the base to a point 2 cm caudal to the atrioventricular sulcus leaving the atrioventricular apparatus intact. Cross sections of the heart can be evaluated for dilation (dilated cardiomyopathy, DCM) or hypertrophy. Consideration of a diagnosis of hypertrophic cardiomyopathy requires that the LV is hypertrophied in the absence of a systemic or primary cardiac cause (i.e., hyperthyroidism or hypertension). In cats, the distribution of hypertrophy may be segmental instead of diffuse HCM (HCM phenotypes Fig. 6.6). The heart base/atrioventricular apparatus is then dissected according to the flow of blood, beginning in the right atrium as before. Alternatively, the right ventricular outflow tract can be opened and then cut retrograde through the right AV valve into the right atrium close to the septum.

Tomographic dissection allows for dissection of the heart along standard echocardiographic views and enhances correlation and sampling of specific lesions noted during imaging (Fig. 6.6). The heart can be sectioned along a long axis 4 chamber plane or a long axis LV inflow/outflow plane. This method is most easily accomplished using a heart which has already been fixed. For the long axis 4 chamber view, make incisions in the lateral sides and roof of the right and left atria to expose the respective valves. Forceps passed into the valve orifices serve as guides for a very sharp blade to section the heart from base to apex. For the LV inflow/outflow plane, forceps to guide the cut would be inserted in the MV orifice and aorta.

Whenever possible, the entire heart should be submitted for examination and sampling by a pathologist. Should this not be possible, in addition to sampling lesions, full thickness samples of all chambers of the heart should be submitted in 10% neutral buffered formalin for the evaluation of microscopic disease. These samples include right ventricular free wall, interventricular septum, sections of both left ventricular papillary muscles, and left ventricular outflow tract; all samples should be taken from the middle third of the of the chambers. In cats in particular, multiple samples of left ventricular outflow track are recommended. Samples of the right ventricular anterolateral and the outflow tract free wall should be sampled if boxer cardiomyopathy/arrhythmogenic right ventricular cardiomyopathy is suspected. Alternatively, a "T" cut to include the left ventricular free wall, interventricular septum, and the right ventricular free wall as well as a section of the IVS parallel to the outflow track that includes the septal leaflet of the right atrioventricular valve and left ventricular outflow tract can be taken. Cardiac disease in small animals frequently has a familial or inherited component; in a small percentage of these diseases, genetic tests for specific mutations using EDTA blood, splenic tissue or cheek swabs may be available.

In cases where precise sampling of the conduction system is required to exclude or document conduction system abnormalities, it is strongly suggested to send the whole heart to a lab with an experienced cardiopathologist. In most species, it is difficult to identify and consistently obtain adequate samples of the conduction system even with extensive knowledge of the landmarks. In addition, it is difficult to interpret subtle degenerative changes (fibrosis, age-related changes) in the sinoatrial node and atrioventricular node.

6.4 Common Artifacts, Non-lesions, and Postmortem Changes

The supporting architecture of the heart is robust and thus the heart is less prone to some of the artifacts related to autolysis.

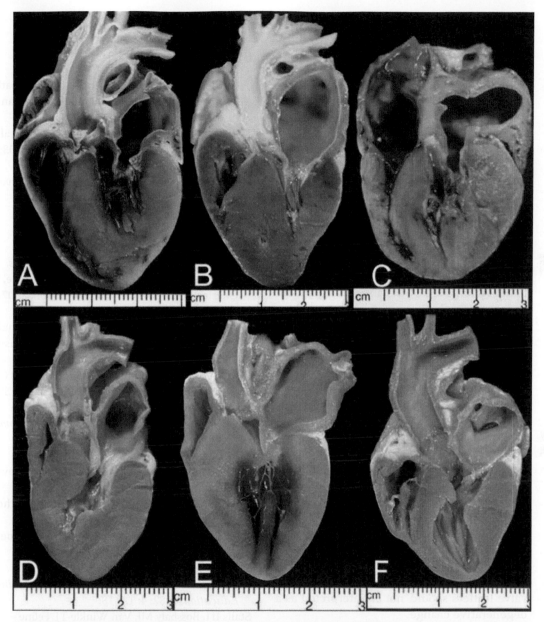

Figure 6.6 Long axis LV inflow/outflow (A, B, D, E, F) and five chamber (C) tomographic sections of hearts from cats with hypertrophic cardiomyopathy (HCM). Distribution of hypertrophy in cats includes both segmental (E-F) and diffuse (A-D). Figure reprinted from *Journal of Veterinary Cardiology*, 5/2, Philip R. Fox, Hypertrophic Cardiomyopathy. Clinical and Pathologic Correlates, Pages 39–45, Copyright (2003), with permission from Elsevier.

1) Barbiturate solution. An iridescent to crystalline to chalky precipitate can be observed lining the epicardial or endocardial surface of the heart of euthanized animals (see Fig. 2.11). In addition, soft tan foci resembling necrosis can be observed in the myocardium of animals euthanized by intracardiac puncture; these artifacts are

associated with a chemical odor. Euthanasia solution can change the clotted blood within the heart, especially in the right ventricle, to a thick, pasty, tan coagulum with the same medicinal odor. Hemorrhage may be observed within the pericardium and thorax as a consequence of intrathoracic or intracardiac puncture.

2) Epicardial, myocardial, and endocardial hemorrhage are common postmortem findings which, in may cases, represent agonal change rather than significant cardiac disease.

3) Hemoglobin imbibition. Given the intimate contact with blood, the heart and vessels readily take up hemoglobin pigment from lysed red cells. This is primarily restricted to the endocardium but can be transmural in the great vessels.

4) Valve edema. Variable valvular thickening of no significance can be observed affecting any of the valves (particularly the right AV). Edematous valves appear gelatinous due to accumulation of clear watery fluid while myxomatous valve disease is characterized by variably coalescing opaque nodular aggregates most evident at the free edge of valve leaflets.

5) Epicardial fat. Well demarcated areas of adipose may occur within the epicardium.

6) Differentiating antemortem from postmortem blood clots. The heart and vessels usually contain postmortem clotted blood which may interdigitate with the chamber trabeculations and give the false impression of attachment.

7) Nodules of Arantius of the aortic semilunar valve leaflets should not be interpreted as a degenerative change.

8) The thickness of the right and left ventricular walls are approximately equal in the neonate.

9) High heart weight to body weight ratio in athletic animals represents physiologic and not pathologic hypertrophy.

Bibliography

Basso C, Fox PR, Meurs KM, et al. Arrhythmogenic right ventricular cardiomyopathy causing sudden cardiac death in boxer dogs: a new animal model of human disease. *Circulation* 2004; 109: 1180–1185.

Fox PR. Hypertrophic cardiomyopathy. Clinical and pathologic correlates. *J Vet Cardiol* 2003; 5: 39–45.

Fox PR. Endomyocardial fibrosis and restrictive cardiomyopathy: pathologic and clinical features. *J Vet Cardiol* 2004; 6: 25–31.

King JM, Roth-Johnson L, Newson ME. *The Necropsy Book: A Guide for Veterinary Students, Residents, Clinicians, Pathologists, and Biological Researchers*. 5th edn. Gurnee, Ill: Charles Louis Davis, DVM Foundation, 2007.

Kittleson MD, Meurs KM, Munro MJ, et al. Familial hypertrophic cardiomyopathy in maine coon cats: an animal model of human disease. *Circulation* 1999; 99:3 172–3180.

Liu SK. Postmortem examination of the heart. *Vet Clin North Am Small Anim Pract* 1983; 13: 379–394.

Meurs KM. Genetics of cardiac disease in the small animal patient. *Vet Clin North Am Small Anim Pract* 2010; 40: 701–715.

Miller ME, Evans HE, DeLahunta A. *Miller's Anatomy of the Dog*. 4th edn. St. Louis: Elsevier Saunders, 2013.

Palate BM, Denoel SR, Roba JL. A simple method for performing routine histopathological examination of the cardiac conduction tissue in the dog. *Toxicol Pathol* 1995; 23: 56–62.

Roth LR KJ. Nonlesions and lesion of no significance. *The Compendium on Continuing Education*, 1982; 4: 13–18.

Stalis IH, Bossbaly MJ, Van Winkle TJ. Feline endomyocarditis and left ventricular endocardial fibrosis. *Vet Pathol* 1995; 32: 122–126.

Turk JR RC. Necropsy of the canine heart: a simple technique for quantifying ventricular hypertrophy and valvular alterations. *Compend Contin Educ Pract Vet* 1983; 5: 905–910.

7

The Respiratory System

7.1 Anatomy Review

The respiratory system is functionally divided into two parts: a conducting system, which conditions and moves air, and an exchange system, which removes carbon dioxide from the blood and replaces it with oxygen. The conduction system consists of the oral and nasal cavities, pharynx, larynx, trachea, bronchi, and proximal bronchioles. The exchange system is composed of respiratory bronchioles, alveoli, alveolar capillaries, and the thin respiratory membrane that separates the alveolar spaces from the capillary lumens. The respiratory system is powered by the skeletal muscle of the diaphragm, which is innervated by the phrenic nerve. The phrenic nerve arises from C5–7 in dogs and C4–7 in cats. A group of nuclei in the brainstem (including the nucleus tractus solitarius and nucleus ambiguous) drive the contraction and relaxation of the diaphragm, as well as coordinating muscles of the tongue, pharynx, and larynx.

The nasal cavity (Fig. 7.1) extends from the nares to the cribriform plate of the ethmoid bone and is bordered dorsally by the maxilla and palatine process of the incisive bone and ventrally by the hard palate. A septum, which is caudally continuous with the ethmoid bone and more rostrally composed of hyaline cartilage, separates the left and right portions of the nasal cavity. Much of the cavity is filled by delicate scrolls of turbinate bones, arranged into rostral (dorsal, middle, and ventral) and caudal (ethmoidal) conchae. The conchae define three passageways for air flow through the nasal cavities: the dorsal, middle, and ventral meatuses. These bones are covered by respiratory epithelium and aid in warming, filtering and humidifying inspired air and directing inhaled pheromones and odorants to the vomeronasal organ and olfactory epithelium.

The maxillary and frontal sinuses are air filled spaces within the skull bones that are lined by respiratory epithelium and communicate with the nasal cavity. In the dog, the maxillary sinus is referred to as the maxillary recess because of the large connection with the nasal cavity.

The pharynx is divided by the soft palate into the oropharynx and nasopharynx. The larynx connects the pharynx to the trachea and consists of three unpaired (epiglottic, thyroid, and cricoid) and one paired (arytenoid) cartilages. The epiglottic cartilage is composed of a stalk, which is attached to the base of the tongue, the basihyoid bones and the body of the thyroid cartilage, and a flexible blade, which curves toward the soft palate at rest, but tilts caudodorsally during swallowing to partially cover the entrance to the larynx. The thyroid cartilage, the largest cartilage in the larynx, is "V" shaped and forms the bulk of the laryngeal floor. The cricoid cartilage is ring shaped and is the most caudal part of the larynx. The paired arytenoid cartilages are triangular and have vocal processes which project into the laryngeal lumen and serve as the attachment site for the vocal folds. The intrinsic muscles of the larynx are the crycothyroideus, crycoarytenoideus

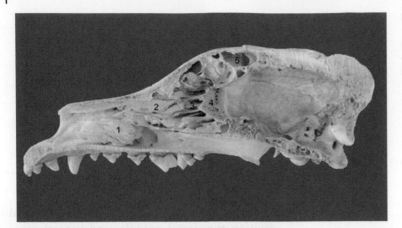

Figure 7.1 The canine nasal cavity. 1. Ventral nasal concha; 2. Dorsal nasal concha; 3. Ethmoidal conchae; 4. Cribriform plate; 5. Frontal sinus.

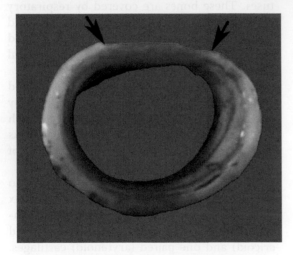

Figure 7.2 Cross section of the canine trachea. The incomplete cartilaginous rings are joined by the dorsal tracheal ligament (arrows).

dorsalis and lateralis, thryoarytenoideus, and arytenoideus transversus.

The hyoid apparatus supports the larynx and the base of the tongue (see Fig. 5.4). This structure consists of four paired and one unpaired bones: the thyrohyoids, which articulate with the thyroid cartilage; the keratohyoids; the epihyoids; the stylohyoids, which articulate with connect to the base of the skull via the tympanohyoid cartilages; and the unpaired basihyoid, which connects the left and right sides of the hyoid apparatus.

The trachea and bronchi conduct air between the larynx and the lung parenchyma. The rigidity of the trachea is provided by "C"-shaped strips of cartilage which are joined along the dorsal aspect by the trachealis muscle, or dorsal tracheal ligament, to form tracheal rings (Fig. 7.2). Inside the rings is a submucosa rich in mucous glands lined by a pseudostratified to simple columnar epithelium. In the distal, small bronchi, the cartilage rings are often replaced by irregularly-shaped plates of cartilage. Bronchioles, in contrast, have smooth muscle rather than cartilage in the walls and are lined by simple cuboidal epithelium. Bronchioles form the transition zone between the conducting and gas exchange parts of the respiratory system. Distal bronchioles, or respiratory bronchioles, are capable of gas exchange; however, the bulk of gas exchange occurs in the sac like terminal alveoli.

The lungs are divided into lobes based on the branching pattern of the primary bronchi (Fig. 7.3). The hilus of the lung is the medial area where the mainstem bronchi and vessels enter the pulmonary parenchyma. The lungs have two separate blood supplies: unoxygenated blood flows to the lungs from the right ventricle via the pulmonary artery and oxygenated blood arrives through the bronchial arteries, which are branches off the thoracic aorta. Both cats and dogs have a right lung that is subdivided into four lobes: cranial, middle, caudal, and

Figure 7.3 The canine airways, ventral view. 1. Trachea; 2. Left mainstem bronchus; 3. Right mainstem bronchus; 4. Bronchus to cranial part of the left cranial lung lobe; 5. Bronchus to caudal part of the left cranial lung lobe; 6. Bronchus to left caudal lung lobe; 7. Bronchus to right cranial lung lobe; 8. Bronchus to right middle lung lobe; 9. Bronchus to right caudal lung lobe; 10. Bronchus to right accessory lung lobe.

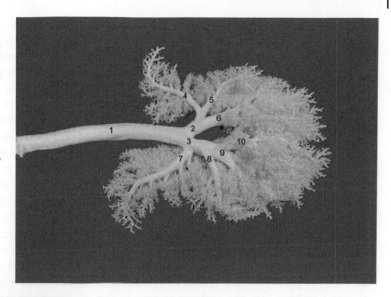

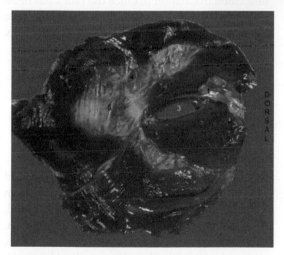

Figure 7.4 Anatomy of the diaphragm, cranial view. 1. Aorta; 2. Crura; 3. Esophageal hiatus; 4. Opening for caudal vena cava; 5. Central tendon.

accessory; and a left lung that is subdivided into two lobes: cranial (with a cranial and caudal part) and caudal. The surface of the lungs is covered by a layer of mesothelium called the visceral pleura, and a similar mesothelial layer, the parietal pleura, lines the inside of the thoracic cavity and diaphragm. The space between the two layers of mesothelium is the pleural cavity. In a normal animal, this is more of a potential space, containing only a few milliliters of clear serous lubricating fluid. Negative pressure in the thoracic cavity maintains close apposition between the visceral and parietal layers and prevents collapse of the lungs.

The diaphragm arises from the cranial lumbar vertebrae as thick bands of muscle called the left and right crura, which fan out and attach to the medial surface of the caudal ribs and the sternum (Fig. 7.4). The center of the diaphragm is tendinous, while the periphery is composed of muscle fibers. The aorta and esophagus transverse the muscular portion of the diaphragm at the dorsal midline, while the caudal vena cava passes through the right side of the tendinous portion.

7.2 *In Situ* Evaluation and Removal

As with all body systems, the respiratory system is examined in a systematic, consistent manner. Begin with an external examination, evaluating the nasal planum, nares, and external contour of the nasal cavity for size, symmetry, discharges, or discoloration. Palpate along the neck and the thoracic wall for any abnormalities. Begin initial examination of the internal structures once the skin, subcutaneous tissues, lateral cervical muscles, and limbs have been reflected from the right side of the body. Reflection of the soft tissues along the lateral neck and jaw exposes the trachea, and reflection of the tissues overlying the right lateral chest allows examination of the ribs, sternum, intercostal muscles, and thoracic inlet. Lesions such a fractures, masses, and hemorrhages may become obvious at this time.

Examine the diaphragm once the abdominal cavity is opened, but prior to opening the thoracic cavity. When viewed from the abdominal side, the diaphragm should be convex and taut. Reach under the ribs, and puncture the diaphragm at the highest point, near the insertion onto the last right rib, creating a full thickness slit into the pleural cavity. In a fresh carcass, this causes a sudden loss of negative pressure in the thorax, leading to an audible rush of air into the cavity and the diaphragm becomes flaccid. Failure to observe this loss of negative pressure can indicate the presence of thoracic lesions, or may be a result of autolysis; thus, this finding should be interpreted in the context of the overall condition of the carcass.

Extend the diaphragmatic incision and check for fluid in the thoracic cavity. If fluid is present, a sample can be collected aseptically for culture and/or cytology. To measure the volume of fluid in the thorax, use a syringe to collect the fluid which is easily accessible at this point, and collect the rest once the thoracic cavity is opened. Use your knife or scalpel to completely detach the right side of the diaphragm from the last right rib and the sternum.

Removal of the right side of the rib cage is accomplished by cutting the ribs at the level of the costo-vertebral and costo-sternal joints. Begin with the last rib and cut towards the thoracic inlet. As the ribcage is removed, the right thoracic cavity is examined for adhesions between the visceral and parietal pleura, presence and character of effusions, and any abnormalities to the chest wall.

After the ribs have been removed, the respiratory tract can be evaluated *in situ*, noting the size, location, anatomic organization, and proportions of the organs in context of the size and conformation of the animal. Once removed from the body, it is more difficult to judge the proportions of the organs. Collect any remaining fluid in the pleural cavity, and note the degree to which the lungs fill the space, as well as their color and contour. Normal lungs, in a fresh carcass should be soft and pink, with a smooth, shiny surface and no rib impressions or adhesions to the thoracic wall or diaphragm. The lungs should collapse slightly when the thoracic cavity is opened, but continue to fill the majority of the thoracic cavity.

The respiratory tract is removed from the body along with the esophagus, thyroid glands, heart, mediastinal structures, and the thoracic vasculature (collectively known as the pluck) as described in Chapter 3. Once the pluck has been removed, examine the left side of the thoracic cavity and pleura, and collect and quantify any remaining fluid.

7.3 Organ Examination, Sectioning, and Fixation

7.3.1 Larynx and Trachea

The larynx and trachea should be evaluated after the esophagus and pharynx have been either separated or opened and examined. Examine the length and contour of the trachea. Dorsoventral flattening of the tracheal rings, with widening of the dorsal longitudinal ligament, can be indicative of cartilage degeneration (associated with the clinical syndrome of tracheal collapse), and tracheal hypoplasia with decreased diameter of the tracheal rings is also part of brachycephalic airway syndrome.

Before opening the larynx, observe the external musculature for evidence of asymmetry, atrophy, inflammation or other abnormalities. Open the larynx and trachea by cutting along the dorsal midline, through the trachealis muscle, with a knife or scissors. In large dogs, bone cutting forceps may be required to cut through the laryngeal cartilage. Avoid running instruments or fingers along the mucosa of any sections that will be submitted for histology, as this will disrupt the mucosal epithelium. Extend the incision into the primary and lobar bronchi. The normal tracheal and bronchial mucosa is smooth, glistening, and pale white to pink. The lumina of the trachea and bronchioles may contain a small amount of frothy white to pink fluid. Abundant tracheal fluid or foam may suggest pulmonary edema, but should always be interpreted in conjunction with evaluation of the pulmonary parenchyma. Blood, thick mucus, ingesta, or foreign material in the trachea is abnormal.

Samples for histopathology should include representative full thickness samples of the trachea, including the cartilage. In cats and small dogs, a good section for histology is one that includes the base of the tongue, larynx, and proximal trachea and esophagus. In large dogs, these tissues may need to be separated for fixation. A fresh sample of the trachea may also be saved for infectious disease testing if the history or gross findings indicate.

7.3.2 Lungs

The lungs are evaluated visually and via light palpation prior to sectioning. Except in special cases, the lungs are best evaluated after the heart has been removed. The presence of rib impressions on the pleural surface, failure of the parenchyma to collapse and alterations in color and texture can indicate abnormalities. The color of lungs depends on a variety of factors, including the thickness of the pleura, the relative amount of gas and blood in the tissue, and the degree of postmortem autolysis (see Section 7.5). In general, the color of the lungs should only be relied upon as an indication of pulmonary disease in a fresh carcass. Changes in lung texture and compliance are much more reliable indications of disease.

Atelectatic areas are dark red to purple and collapsed. Animals that die while breathing 100% oxygen will have diffusely atelectic lungs because the oxygen can be completely absorbed,

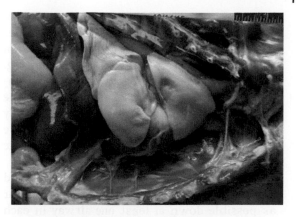

Figure 7.5 Pale pink lungs from an anemic puppy.

unlike inhaled room air which contains 78% nitrogen. Fetuses and stillborn animals will also have atelectic lungs. Diffuse dark red discoloration of lungs that are well aerated usually indicates congestion, while multifocal discrete areas of dark red discoloration suggest pulmonary hemorrhage. Pale tan to white lungs suggest anemia or severe blood loss (Fig. 7.5). In cases of heart failure, lungs may have a subtle brown tinge due to the presence of hemosiderin.

Palpation is done gently, so as not to jeopardize the quality of the sample for histopathology. Palpation can aid in detection of masses not obvious from the surface, or changes in consistency. Interpretation of pulmonary texture requires practice, palpating many normal and abnormal lungs. In general, normal lungs are slightly spongy and subtly crepitent. Factors such the age of the animal, and postmortem interval can alter this texture. Old dogs often have areas of osseous metaplasia in the lung, which will be palpable as small, gritty foci. Pulmonary texture can be classified as rubbery (edema, atelectasis, or postmortem collapse), firm (inflammatory or neoplastic infiltrate) or hard (mineralized). However, differentiating between a rubbery lung, indicative of edema, atelectasis, or postmortem collapse, and a firm lung with interstitial pneumonia can be difficult; histologic examination is often required for a definitive diagnosis.

Full assessment of lung lesions includes an estimate of the percent of lung or lung lobes affected, as well as evaluation of the distribution (focal, multifocal, multifocal to coalescing, locally extensive, or diffuse) and pattern (random, dorsocaudal, or cranioventral) of the changes. Bacterial bronchopneumonia typically affects the cranioventral lung lobes while diffuse or dorsocaudal distribution is more characteristic of a viral interstitial pneumonia.

The cuts into the mainstem bronchi should be extended, using blunt-tipped scissors, as far as possible down at least one airway in each lung to look for foreign material, excessive mucus, blood, or parasites. Once the airways have been explored, the lungs should be serially sectioned ("bread-loafed") with a very sharp knife, using long smooth cuts, avoiding crushing the tissue. Variation in texture, exudates, hemorrhages and some masses may only be evidenced on sectioning. Also, a significant amount of fluid oozing from the cut surfaces of the sections is strongly suggestive of pulmonary edema.

Samples of lung for histopathology should include sections of each lung lobe, including at least one section from the periphery of the lobe and one from near the hilus, as well as sections of all lesions. For large lesions, a sample from the periphery which includes some adjacent normal tissue is usually preferred (sections from the center of a mass may be completely necrotic and of little histologic value). Because lung tissue is so malleable, collection of thin sections can be a challenge; fortunately, the airspaces in the tissue enable formalin fixation, so samples will fix adequately even if they slightly exceed the 1 cm limit imposed for other histopathology samples. Lung samples should float when placed into formalin; failure to do so (except in a fetus or stillborn animal) is indicative of abnormal aeration. If samples are to be submitted for ancillary testing, they should be collected aseptically, prior to extensive manipulation. Given that some infectious diseases can be multifactorial, testing for both viral and bacterial agents is often indicated.

7.3.3 Nasal Cavity and Sinuses

Examination of the nasal cavities and sinuses is easiest after the brain has been removed. The frontal sinuses are often opened with the transverse cut through the skull during brain removal. Bone cutting forceps can be used to chip away the remaining frontal bone and permit a clear view into the cavity. The sinuses should contain only air, so any fluid or other material is a significant finding. The nasal cavity is opened and examined by using a saw to either create serial transverse sections through the cavities or by splitting it longitudinally on the midline. The former method is best for evaluating symmetry of the internal nasal structures, and also allows examination of the maxillary sinuses, while the latter technique provides better exposure of the nasal septum, extent of the nasal cavities and evaluation of the cribriform plate.

Samples of sinus or nasal cavity bone and mucosa for histology can be collected using bone cutting forceps (to collect some bone fragments with mucosa) or an oscillating saw (to collect a thin slice of bone and mucosa). Most samples will require decalcification prior to histologic processing.

7.4 Special Techniques

If indicated (suspected pulmonary embolism), the pulmonary vasculature can also be opened. At the hilus of each lung, adjacent to the mainstem bronchus, locate the left and right branches of the pulmonary artery, and use blunt-tipped scissors to open the arteries to look for thrombi or parasites.

In small animals, the lungs can be insufflated with formalin to inflate the alveoli for rapid fixation and optimal histopathology sections. A technique for lung insufflation is described in Chapter 15.

Lungs can also be inflated, using any available source of air. The tube is sealed to the cut trachea using string or a zip tie. Inflating the lungs can identify ruptured bullae, which may be the cause of pneumothorax.

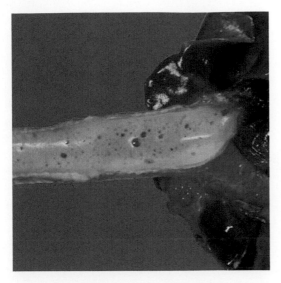

Figure 7.6 Foam in the trachea is a common postmortem finding, and is considered an artifact unless the lungs are also wet and heavy, consistent with pulmonary edema.

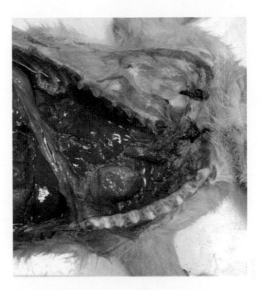

Figure 7.7 The color and consistency of lungs changes dramatically with prolonged postmortem intervals. The lungs in this animal are dark red and collapsed secondary to postmortem autolysis rather than respiratory disease.

7.5 Common Artifacts and Postmortem Changes

1) Foam in the trachea and airways (Fig. 7.6). While this finding may be suggestive of pulmonary edema, foam can also develop secondary to euthanasia or agonal breathing. Interpretation of this finding should take into consideration other gross findings (such as fluid oozing from cut surface of the lung), as well as clinical history and radiographic findings.

2) Variation in lung color. As the lungs are very vascular, and their bulk is primarily due to the presence of air in the tissue, the appearance of the lungs can vary greatly as the postmortem interval increases. Blood pools in the lungs and pulmonary gasses diffuse into the environment, causing the lungs to become mottled, wet, shrunken, heavy, and rubbery (Fig. 7.7). Blood will settle predominantly in the dependent lung (livor mortis).

Bibliography

Dyce KM, Sack WO, Wensing CJG. 1996. *Textbook of Veterinary Anatomy*, 2nd edn, pp. 151–168, 403–408. Philadelphia, PA: WB Saunders Company.

Evans HE, de Lahunta, A. 2012. *Miller's Anatomy of the Dog*, 4th edn. New York: Elsevier, electronic edition.

King JM, Roth-Johnson L, Newson, ME. 2007. *The Necropsy Book: A Guide for Veterinary Students, Residents, Clinicians, Pathologists, and Biological Researchers.* 5th edn. Gurnee, Ill.: Charles Louis Davis, DVM Foundation.

Maxie, M Grant. 2015. In *Jubb, Kennedy and Palmer's Pathology of Domestic Animals*, Vol. 2, 6th edn. New York: Saunders Elsevier.

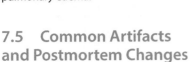

Common Artifacts and Postmortem Changes

Foam in the trachea and airways (Fig. 7.6). While this finding may be suggestive of pulmonary edema, foam can also develop secondary to euthanasia or agonal breathing. Interpretation of this finding should take into consideration other gross findings (such as fluid oozing from cut surface of the lung), as well as clinical history and radiographic findings.

Variation in lung color. As the lungs are very vascular, and their bulk is primarily due to the presence of air in the tissue, the appearance of the lungs can vary greatly as the postmortem interval increases. Blood pools in the lungs and pulmonary gasses diffuse into the environment, causing the lungs to become mottled, wet, shrunken, heavy, and rubbery (Fig. 7.7). Blood will settle predominantly in the dependent lung (livor mortis).

Figure 7.6 Foam in the trachea is a common postmortem finding, and is considered an artifact unless the lungs are also wet and heavy, consistent with pulmonary edema.

Figure 7.7 The color and consistency of lungs changes dramatically with prolonged postmortem intervals. The lungs in this animal are dark red and collapsed secondary to postmortem autolysis rather than respiratory disease.

Bibliography

Dyce KM, Sack WO, Wensing CJG. 1996. Textbook of Veterinary Anatomy, 2nd edn, pp 151-168, 404-408. Philadelphia, PA: WB Saunders Company.

Evans HE, de Lahunta, A. 2012. Miller's Anatomy of the Dog, 4th edn. New York: Elsevier, electronic edition.

King JM, Roth-Johnson L, Newson ME. 2005. The Necropsy Book: A Guide for Veterinary Students, Residents, Clinicians, Pathologists, and Biological Researchers, 6th edn. Gurnee, IL: Charles Louis Davis, DVM Foundation.

Maxie, M G (ed). 2015. In Jubb, Kennedy, and Palmer's Pathology of Domestic Animals, Vol. 2, 6th ed. New York: Saunders Elsevier.

8

The Alimentary System

8.1 Anatomy Review

The alimentary system consists of a long and convoluted tube together with several associated structures that are primarily responsible for uptake, digestion, and absorption of nutrients, but also for immune protection against invaders and maintenance of homeostasis. The alimentary tract begins at one end of the body with the mouth or oropharyngeal cavity and ends at the other end with the anus.

The oropharyngeal cavity is a complex structure involved in prehension, mastication and deglutition of food and water; however, it is also essential for defense, hunting, and play. From there, the ingesta transits rapidly through the dorsal thoracic cavity, across the diaphragm and into the stomach, by way of the esophagus, a relatively simple muscular tube. The ingesta is temporarily stored in the stomach where it undergoes the first phase of the digestive process before proceeding through the small intestine where digestive enzymes and bile, respectively secreted by the pancreas and gall bladder, are added to allow for more complete digestion and absorption of nutrients. Unabsorbed contents including secretory products and water reach the cecum and colon before passing through the pelvic canal and exiting at the anus. Associated with the alimentary system is a large complement of lymphoid structures that are involved in innate and adaptive immune defenses. These structures range from well-developed tonsils in the pharynx and organized lymph nodes along the length of the alimentary tract to mucosa-associated lymphoid aggregates and Peyer's patches of the intestine interconnected by a network of lymphatic vessels.

8.1.1 The Oropharyngeal Cavity

The oropharyngeal cavity consists of the lips which are continuous with the oral and gingival mucosa that covers the inner surfaces of the cheeks, and surrounds the teeth. The tongue occupies the ventral aspect of the oral cavity, while the rostral hard plate and caudal soft palate are along the roof. The caudal pharyngeal space directs air from the nasopharynx into the larynx and food and water from the oropharynx into the esophagus. The mucosa lining these structures contains the paired palatine tonsils and auditory tubes. Within the tissues surrounding the pharynx and neck are several salivary glands and lymph nodes.

The tongue is composed of skeletal muscle covered by a relatively smooth mucous membrane in the dog. In the cat, the tongue is covered by a thick brush-like layer composed of filiform papilla with a caudally oriented keratinized spine important for grooming. The palatine tonsils are relatively small in the cat, less than 0.3 cm, while in the dog, they vary according to body size and can range from 1.0 × 0.4 cm up to 2.0 × 1.0 cm in a large dog. In both the dog and the cat, they are located on either side of the pharynx just cranial to the larynx. They are covered by a semilunar fold and hidden in a deep fossa.

Necropsy Guide for Dogs, Cats, and Small Mammals, First Edition. Edited by Sean P. McDonough and Teresa Southard.
© 2017 John Wiley & Sons, Inc. Published 2017 by John Wiley & Sons, Inc.
Companion Website: www.wiley.com/go/mcdonough/necropsy

The teeth are highly mineralized structures that are essential for cutting and crushing food, but also for defense, hunting, and play. The number and type of permanent teeth can be expressed by the formula 2 (Incisor 3/3 – Canine 1/1 - Pre-molar 4/4 – Molar 2/3) = 42 for the dog, and 2 (Incisor 3/3 – Canine 1/1 - Pre-molar 3/2 – Molar 1/1) = 30 for the cat. However, the modified Triadan System for the dog and the cat (Floyd, 1991) is a more accurate and universal method for numbering teeth during gross necropsy (see Fig. 5.5).

8.1.2 The Salivary Glands

The salivary glands consist of multiple paired secretory units that include major and minor components. There are four major salivary glands in the dog and the cat; the parotid, mandibular, sublingual, and zygomatic glands. The cat also has molar salivary glands. These glands are well-circumscribed, encapsulated, multilobulated units that are separated by thin connective tissue septa each with their own separate excretory duct. By contrast, minor salivary glands are composed of microscopic clusters of secretory units named according to their location in the oral submucosa; labial, lingual (between muscle bundles of the tongue), buccal, palatine, and pharyngeal. Only the major salivary glands are examined grossly; however, they can be difficult to distinguish from lymph nodes located in the same area. The parotid and mandibular salivary glands are uniformly pale yellow to tan, while the sublingual glands are pink to light red. On the cut surface, salivary tissue consists of small lobules divided by thin linear bands of connective tissue. By contrast, lymph nodes are generally uniformly light yellow to dark red, and on section, have a distinct outer homogeneous to slightly nodular whitish cortex with a darker pink to light red slightly depressed central medullary region. On section, the cortex of lymph nodes bulges and the medulla oozes clear yellow to pink fluid.

The parotid salivary glands are slightly nodular and irregular structures located within the subcutaneous tissues at the back of the vertical ramus of the mandibular bones. These glands have a deep V-shaped indentation that closely wraps around the base of each ear. Ventral and slightly caudal and medial to the parotid salivary glands are the larger mandibular salivary glands. In a large dog, they can be 5 cm in length and 3 cm wide. There are two to four mandibular lymph nodes located just cranial to each of the mandibular salivary glands. Caudal and more medial to the mandibular salivary glands and extending under the sternomastoideus muscle are the medial retropharyngeal lymph nodes. The sublingual salivary glands consist of two distinct portions. A monostomatic (compact) component lies close to the cranial medial aspect of the mandibular gland and extends cranially for a few centimeters toward the base of the tongue. The polystomatic (diffuse) portion of the sublingual gland extends further rostrally under the oral mucosa within the sublingual fold besides the frenulum of the tongue. The zygomatic salivary glands are located below the eyes, deep under the zygomatic arch. The molar salivary glands of the cat have an elongated rectangular shape, and are located in the fascia beneath the mucosa of the lower lip near the oral commissures, forming a 7 mm irregular bulge lingual to the mandibular molar.

8.1.3 The Esophagus

The esophagus is a tubular organ that joins the pharynx to the stomach. It opens dorsal to the larynx at the pharyngoesophageal lumen, a circumferential plication of the mucosa that forms a shallow ridge. The cervical portion of the esophagus extends along the neck, dorsal to the trachea, and passes through the thoracic inlet into the thoracic cavity. The thoracic part of the esophagus lies to the left of the trachea at the thoracic inlet and extends dorsally to the trachea in the thoracic cavity. Within the thorax, it lies above the heart with the aortic arch on the left before passing through the esophageal hiatus where it joins the stomach at the cardia to

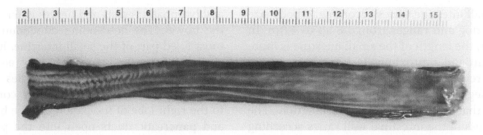

Figure 8.1 Opened esophagus of an adult cat with prominent shallow circumferential ridges imparting a herring-bone pattern to the distal one-third of the mucosal surface.

the left of the medial plane and ventral to thoracic vertebra 11–12. Running along most of the length of the outer muscle layer of the esophagus are the right and left vagal nerves which divide into ventral and dorsal branches just past the base of the heart near the tracheobronchial lymph node. The right and left ventral branches unite to form the ventral vagal trunk, while the dorsal vagal trunk joins further caudally. The mucosa of the esophagus has longitudinal folds and is uniformly smooth in the dog, while in the cat, the distal one-third of the esophagus has shallow circumferential ridges that impart a herring-bone appearance to the mucosal surface (Fig. 8.1).

Submucosal glands are present throughout the esophagus from the pharyngoesophageal junction to the cardia in the dog, while they are present only in the cervical portion near the pharyngoesophageal junction in the cat. The outer tunica muscularis layer of the esophagus is composed of striated muscle the entire length of the esophagus in the dog, while in the cat only the cranial two-thirds to four-fifths is composed of striated muscle with the caudal one-third to one-fifth consisting of smooth muscle.

8.1.4 The Stomach

The stomach is an eccentric sac-like dilation of the proximal intestinal tract owing to a lesser curvature that is approximately four times shorter than the greater curvature. It lays in the left lateral quadrant of the abdominal cavity, caudal to the liver and separated from the left

abdominal wall by the spleen. The body of the stomach bulges ventrally, caudal to the left costal arch along the abdominal wall halfway between the xiphoid cartilage and the pubis. The mucosa consists of a short cardia followed by a wide fundus and body that extends to the right as a narrower cylindrical pylorus before opening into the duodenum at the pyloric opening. The wall of the stomach consists of a thick smooth muscle layer surrounding the submucosa and mucosa. When the stomach is full, the mucosa is relatively flat; however, when empty it has prominent folds or rugae. The thickness of the stomach wall is approximately 3–5 mm in the dog, while in the cat it ranges from 2 mm between rugae to up to 4.4 mm at the rugae. The capacity of the stomach varies according to body size in the dog and can range from 0.6 up to 8.0 L. The greater omentum is a double-walled sac composed of a meshwork of adipose tissue and vascular structures that extends from the base of the mesentery and attaches along the greater curvature of the stomach forming a large space called the omental bursa. Between the esophagus and the pylorus and along the lesser curvature of the stomach lies one or two small gastric lymph nodes and the lesser omentum.

8.1.5 The Small Intestine

The small intestine fills most of the abdominal cavity from the stomach and liver cranially to the pelvis and urinary bladder caudally. The entire jejunum and ileum are enclosed by the omentum and are connected to the dorsal body wall by the root of the mesentery. The length of the small intestine varies according to body size in the dog and ranges from 1.8 up to 4.8 m. In the cat, the length of the small intestine is more constant and approximately 1.3 m. It is divided into a relatively short duodenum followed by a long segment of jejunum and a short distal ileum that ends at the ileocecal junction. The thickness of the intestinal wall varies according to the segment of intestine and body size in the dog (Table 8.1), while it is relatively uniform in the cat and averages 2.4 mm in the duodenum and 2.1 mm in the jejunum. The entire length of the small intestine is connected to the mesentery along the mesenteric border where blood

Table 8.1 Relative wall thickness (mm) of individual small intestinal segments according to body weight of dog as determined by using ultrasonography.[†]

Segment	Body weight in kg		
	<20	20–40	>40
Duodenum	≤5.1	≤5.3	≤6.0
Jejunum	≤4.1	≤4.4	≤4.7

[†] Modified from: Anderson KL. *Ultrasonography of the GI Tract*, CVM 6105.

and lymphatic vessels and nerves enter and exit the bowel. The descending duodenum is the most fixed part of the small intestine. It begins at the pylorus and runs caudally along the right dorsal abdomen where it lies against the right body wall and is tightly connected to the right lobe of the pancreas. The bile duct and pancreatic ducts open into the proximal duodenum forming small papilla on the mucosal surface. The opening of the bile duct is located approximately 3–8 cm from the pylorus, while the locations of the pancreatic duct openings are variable. The major pancreatic duct is smaller and sometimes absent, but when present, it opens near the bile duct at the major duodenal papilla or hepatopancreatic papilla (ampulla of Vater) located approximately 7.5 cm from the pylorus (Fig. 8.5). The accessory pancreatic duct is larger and opens into the minor duodenal papilla located 6–13 cm from the pylorus. Most dogs have major and accessory exocrine pancreatic excretory ducts, while cats have a single major pancreatic duct. In the cat, the hepatic duct fuses with the major pancreatic duct prior to entering the duodenum.

After turning 180 degrees at the caudal duodenal flexure, the ascending duodenum

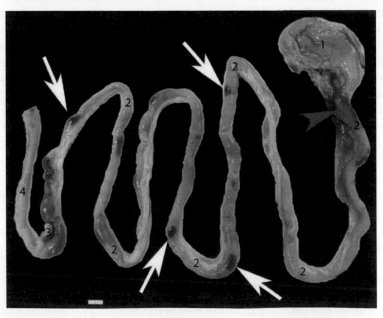

Figure 8.2 Stomach (1), small intestine (2), cecum (3), and colon (4) of a 5-week-old puppy dog with *Ancylostoma caninum* infection. Note the prominent red Peyer's patches on the serosal surface of the small intestine (arrows) and bile imbibition of the descending duodenum (arrow head).

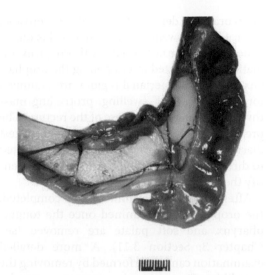

Figure 8.3 Ileocecal junction and cecum of an emaciated 7-week-old cat. Note the small size and sac-like shape of the cecum. The colic lymph nodes are located within the mesentery around the ileocecal junction.

continues along the left side of the root of the mesentery, dorsal to the colon before joining the jejunum at the duodenojejunal flexure. The jejunum is the longest segment of small intestine and occupies most of the ventrocaudal portion of the abdomen. It consists of several loops joined to the dorsal body wall by the mesentery, a variably fatty membrane that contains enteric nerves, blood, and lymphatic vessels along with a chain of anastomosing mesenteric lymph nodes. The distal jejunum connects to the cecum by a short straight segment of ileum. The exact demarcation between the jejunum and ileum is not grossly visible; however, the ileal mucosa of the dog has grossly distinct coalescing submucosal lymphoid aggregates called Peyer's patches (Fig. 8.2). Although the cat has typical Peyer's patches histologically, they are not visible on gross examination. The ileum extends from the left to the right near the midlumbar region caudal to the root of the mesentery where it connects to the cecum and colon at the ileocolic opening (ileocolic valve). The mesentery at the junction between the ileum and cecum contains none to two colic lymph nodes (Fig. 8.3).

8.1.6 The Large Intestine

The large intestine begins at the ileocolic junction and ends at the recto-anal junction. When compared with other animals, the cecum of the dog and the cat are relatively small. It has a separate opening in the colon from the ileocolic opening. In the dog, it consists of a spiral-shaped, blind-end sac (Fig. 8.2), while in the cat, it is much smaller and consists of a short straight blind-end sac (Fig. 8.3). In young dogs, the cecum often has dozens of evenly distributed, sharply demarcated, 0.1 cm up to 0.2 cm in diameter, pale white nodules of lymphoid tissue that are easily seen through the serosal surface. With postmortem decomposition, these nodules can appear from dark grey, black, and even green.

The colon is a relatively straight tube that extends from the cecum to the recto-anal junction and is attached to the sublumbar region by the mesocolon. It has a slightly larger diameter than the small intestine, and in the dog can reach up to 60–75 cm in length. It begins as a short ascending colon that lies medial to the duodenum and right lobe of the pancreas along the right side of the root of the mesentery before turning to the left at the cranial aspect of the root of the mesentery, crossing the medial plane at the right colic flexure to become the transverse colon. The transverse colon then turns caudally at the left colic flexure to become the long descending colon that extends caudally along the medial ventral surface of the left kidney before entering the pelvic inlet in the retroperitoneal space, where it is known as the rectum. The rectum connects to the anus at the recto-anal junction. The small openings of the right and left anal sacs are located on the lateral sides of the recto-anal junction at 2:00 and 10:00 o'clock, respectively. On section, the anal sacs, which are oval and approximately 2–3 cm in the dog, contain a greasy, grey malodorous substance. The recto-anal junction is an epithelial transition zone where the colonic mucosa abruptly changes to anal stratified squamous epithelium.

8.1.7 The Intestinal Vasculature and Nervous System

The arterial blood supply of most of the gastrointestinal tract from the caudal half of the descending duodenum to the cranial part of the descending colon is from the cranial mesenteric artery that originates at the abdominal aorta just cranial to the renal arteries. The stomach and proximal duodenum and pancreas are supplied by branches of the celiac artery; the common hepatic artery, splenic artery, and left gastric artery. The caudal mesenteric artery supplies the mid and caudal portions of the descending colon and cranial portion of the rectum. Arteries and veins travel with lymphatic vessels and nerves through the mesentery and enter or exit the intestine at the mesenteric attachment. The small intestinal circulation of the dog and the cat is unique as it lacks arteriovenous loops. Instead, it has submucosal arteriovenous anastomoses that can shunt blood to the intestinal villi during digestion and open to partially bypass the intestinal villi between digestive periods. The venous return of the stomach, intestine and pancreas enters the portal vein and flows through the liver before returning to the systemic circulation. After leaving the intestine, lymphatic vessels drain into regional lymph nodes before converging through intestinal lymphatic trunks into the cisterna chyli located in the sublumbar region near the crura of the diaphragm. From there, the lymph reaches the thoracic duct and empties into the left brachiocephalic vein. Surrounding the base of the cranial and caudal mesenteric arteries are the cranial and caudal mesenteric plexuses and ganglia.

8.2 *In Situ* Evaluation and Removal

Examination of the alimentary system begins with the lips, oral cavity, anal, and perianal regions as part of the general external examination of the body. If oral or palatal mucosal discoloration, defects (cleft, blister, erosion, ulcer, fistula), swelling, mass, malocclusion, or abnormalities are noted, a more thorough examination is conducted after opening the oropharynx. The anal or perianal regions are examined for the presence of swelling, protruding mass through the anus or prolapse of the rectum. The presence of perianal fecal staining might suggest diarrheal disease. Any abnormalities are noted to direct a more thorough examination to identify the potential underlying cause.

After the external examination is completed, the oropharynx is examined once the tongue, pharynx and soft palate are removed (see Chapter 3, Section 3.11). A more detailed examination can be performed by removing the mandible. First, cut the masseter muscles away from the lateral surface of the angle of the ramus. Do this by inserting the knife at the commissure of the mouth just lateral to the ramus and extend the incision ventrally to the angle of the jaw. Sever the mandibular symphysis with pruning shears or a saw. While pulling back on the mandible, cut the pterygoid muscles behind the last molar. Sever the medial muscular attachments to the medial surface of the ramus and extend the incision around the caudal border of the angle of the mandible. Finally, rotate the mandible laterally to disarticulate the temporomandibular joint and cut any remaining attachments.

The teeth are enumerated and missing or abnormal teeth are recorded by using the modified Triadan System (see Fig. 5.5). The alignment of the jaws (malocclusion) and the presence, degree and distribution of dental deposits (plaque, mineralized calculus/tartar), color, and integrity of the crown (enamel hypoplasia and dysplasia, erosion, fracture, pulp exposure), and exposure, decay, or resorption of the root of the teeth are noted. The color and integrity of the gums, presence of focal or diffuse gingival enlargement or mass, and recession of the gum lines are noted. If warranted, further dissection of the oral structures is described under special techniques at the end of this section.

After examining the surface and underside of the tongue for evidence of mucosal defect or swelling (glossitis, cyst, neoplasia), serial complete transverse sections from the tip to the base of the tongue are made. Changes in color or structural abnormalities within the muscle mass (foreign body, abscess, granuloma, cyst, draining track) are noted. The gums can show evidence of generalized disease process including paleness (anemia), yellow discoloration (icterus), vesicle (<1.0 cm diameter), bulla (>1.0 cm diameter), shallow erosions and ulcers (ruptured vesicle/bulla, viral infection, autoimmune disease, uremia), or local damage (burn, electrocution, chemical, gingivostomatitis, periodontitis).

The tonsils are examined either while still attached to the pharynx together with the pluck or within the pharyngeal area. Finally, the masticatory (masseter, pterigoideus, and temporalis) and pharyngeal musculature and all major salivary glands and local lymph nodes are examined for abnormalities.

8.2.1 The Esophagus

After the thoracic cavity has been opened and before the pluck is removed, the external aspect of the entire length of the esophagus is examined and palpated *in situ* for evidence of external compression (mass, abscess, vascular ring from persistent 4th aortic arch), displacement (hernia, gastroesophageal intussusception), mural enlargement (mass) or narrowing (stricture or stenosis), luminal distention (megaesophagus) or obstruction (foreign body, impaction, mass). The presence of exudate (pyothorax) or feed material in the thoracic cavity should trigger a search for a defect within the wall of the esophagus as a potential underlying cause.

Once the pluck has been removed, the entire length of the esophagus from the pharyngoesophageal lumen to the cardia is opened by using the blunt end of scissors. The lumen should be free of contents, and the presence of dilation, narrowing or partial or complete obstruction should be assessed. The thickness of the wall is evaluated and the mucosa is closely examined for evidence of damage. Animals that have been tube fed might show segmental areas of surface damage including shallow mucosal erosion, ulceration or perforation. Chronic vomiting or regurgitation can cause mucosal damage with or without hyperplasia of lymphoid and glandular tissue characterized by small white nodules mostly along the distal esophageal mucosa.

8.2.2 The Gastrointestinal Tract

Open the abdominal wall (see Chapter 3, Section 3.5). While reflecting the abdominal wall, the presence, volume and appearance of fluid (ascites, blood) or exudate (serous, fibrinous, purulent effusion) in the abdominal cavity is noted. The greater omentum is removed by gentle dissection, while the color, consistency, and presence of nodule or mass is noted. The color, location, and orientation of the abdominal viscera are assessed *in situ* before and after removal of the omentum (Fig. 8.4A and B). Full assessment requires removal of the omentum. On external examination, the normal serosa of the gastrointestinal tract should be light pink to tan with a smooth and shiny surface. Inflammation of the gastrointestinal tract can result in focal to diffuse redness and a diffusely dull serosal surface with a roughened, ground glass appearance. A search for possible extrahepatic shunts is made before disturbing the viscera (see Chapter 9).

The location and extent of external adhesion (peritonitis, previous surgery), compression (mass, abscess, strangulation, pelvic fracture callus), displacement (torsion, volvulus, hernia, sequestration, intussusception), mural enlargement (abscess, granuloma, mass, duplication cyst), plication (linear foreign body), or defect (rupture), luminal narrowing (stricture, stenosis), occlusion (membrane, cord, or blind-end atresia), distention (megacolon, diverticulum), or obstruction (foreign body, impaction, mass) are noted. The presence of ingesta or exudate (peritonitis) in the abdominal cavity should initiate a search for a transmural defect and

(A)

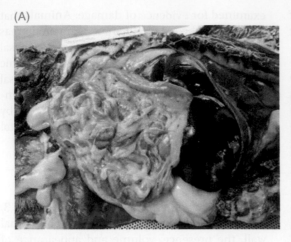

(B)

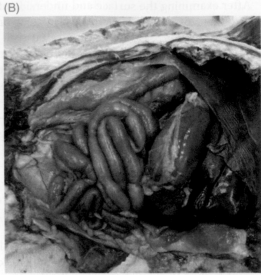

Figure 8.4 Gastrointestinal tract from an adult dog *in situ*. Note the descending duodenum in the right dorsal quadrant of the abdomen and the omentum enclosing the small intestine (removed in B).

leakage. Gastroduodenal perforating ulcers are a common cause of peritonitis in dogs with non-steroidal anti-inflammatory drug toxicity. Gas distention, particularly of the stomach, can lead to rupture and leakage of ingesta in the abdominal cavity; however, this requires careful evaluation in light of the postmortem interval and evidence of antemortem hemorrhage along the margin of a ruptured viscus.

Before removing the intestinal tract from the abdomen, a small incision can be made extending approximately 3–10 cm from the pylorus to expose the major duodenal papilla or hepato-pancreatic papilla (ampulla of Vater). The location of the ampulla can easily be found by gentle compression of the gallbladder to expel bile which also confirms the patency of the bile duct (see Fig. 9.10). Once the external examination is completed, the gastrointestinal tract can be removed *en bloc* and set aside for further examination. This is done by first linearizing the small intestine by incising the mesentery, severing the esophagus at the diaphragm, transecting the distal colon at the pelvic opening, and sectioning the root of the mesentery from the aorta (see Chapter 3: Section 3.12). The spleen is

resected from the greater curvature of the stomach and examined separately (see Chapter 14).

The entire gastrointestinal tract is laid on a cutting board for further assessment (Fig. 8.2). This is facilitated if the small intestine is linearized by cutting the mesentery before removal. As the mesentery is cut, the appearance of the mesenteric vasculature and lymphatic vessels is evaluated for changes in color, tortuosity and presence of nodule or mass. Blood vessels that are more prominent are opened with small sharp-end scissors to assess the presence of obstruction by thromboemboli, or mural abnormalities (vasculitis, neoplasm). In certain forms of protein-losing enteropathy, the mesenteric lymphatic vessels might be more prominent and appear as white, chalky, tortuous tracts (lymphangitis). Additionally in some cases, small, discrete up to 0.5 cm diameter, white, gritty nodules (lipogranulomas) might be scattered along the mesenteric attachment with small white, club-shaped villi along the intestinal mucosa. The serosal surfaces of the stomach and intestines are evaluated for changes in color, texture and segmental or diffuse thickening or increased firmness on palpation.

The intrapelvic segments of the gastrointestinal tract including the distal colon, rectum and anus are removed with the urinary and reproductive organs. Care should be taken not to rupture the anal sacs during removal of these structures. The recto-anal junction should be examined closely for the presence of polypoid mass, particularly in older dogs. Sections of the anal sacs should be collected if there is evidence of inflammation, hemorrhage, necrosis, or a mass.

8.3 Organ Examination, Sectioning, and Fixation

Other than the tongue and tonsils, and unless evidence of a disease process is suspected, other oropharyngeal structures are not routinely sampled for histological examination. The major salivary glands are serially sectioned to look for areas of hemorrhage and necrosis (infarct), fibrosis, cyst, mass, or evidence of inflammation or leakage (sialocele, mucocele). Similarly, the cervical lymph nodes are sectioned and significant enlargement (reactive hyperplasia, neoplasm), abnormal color (hemorrhage, melanin pigment) might indicate drainage of a lesion elsewhere that should initiate further dissection to identify the potential cause. Any nodule or mass is sectioned and the cut surface is assessed to obtain a presumptive diagnosis (abscess, mineral, hematoma, neoplasm).

8.3.1 Gastrointestinal Tract

A complete transverse cross section of the mid-esophagus is routinely taken for fixation and histological assessment. The stomach is opened by making a linear cut starting at the opening of the cardia and extending along the greater curvature following the omental attachment and ending at the gastroduodenal opening by using the blunt end of scissors (Fig. 8.5). After examining the wall for thickness, the volume, composition and consistency of the contents is evaluated. Some contents can be saved for further toxicological analyses. A lack of gastric contents, particularly in neonates or animals with a history of neglect, might suggest reduced feed intake and should be recorded. Abnormal gastric contents, including bile, rocks, carpet fibers, piece of plastic, and so on, might indicate pica and the amount and type should be recorded. In animals with a history of forced-feeding or tube feeding, the volume of gastric contents and whether it is digested or undigested should be noted. The presence of dark red to tarry contents should trigger a search for evidence of mucosal damage (erosion, ulcer, transmural perforation) or neoplasm.

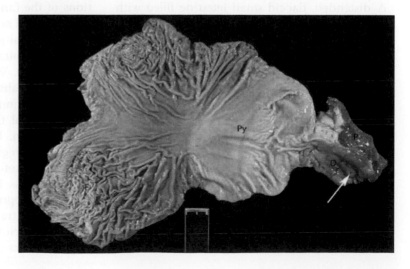

Figure 8.5 Normal stomach including a small portion of the descending duodenum (D) and pancreas (P) of an adult dog. Note the prominent rugae in the fundic mucosa (F) compared with the relatively smooth surfaced pyloric (Py) mucosa. The hepatopancreatic papilla (arrow) is in the descending duodenum. Scale = 2 cm.

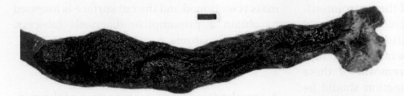

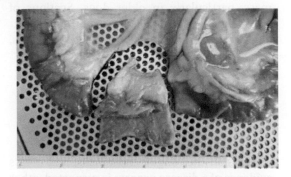

Figure 8.6 Colon of a young adult dog with prominent tarry luminal contents indicative of gastrointestinal bleeding.

The stomach of cats, particularly those with long-hair, often contains some hair. The clinical significance of finding a ball of hair (trichobezoar) in the stomach of a cat is interpreted in light of a history of gastric outflow obstruction, and chronic vomiting.

After examining the mucosa of the fundic and pyloric regions, rectangular sections are taken from each area before removing the contents or washing the mucosa with running water. This allows histological assessment of the mucus layer for the presence of exudate and colonization by various microorganisms. In small dogs, neonatal puppies and kittens, the entire opened stomach can be placed in fixative.

The entire length of the small and large intestine should be opened for complete assessment of the contents and mucosa. The presence, volume and consistency of the contents including foreign materials (toy, stick, string, ear plug, bone, leave, sand, parasites, etc.) are noted. The presence of abnormally watery contents might indicate loss of absorptive function (diarrhea). A distended, flaccid small intestine filled with watery contents and gas might suggest ileus. The presence of undigested blood suggests severe mucosal damage or presence of intestinal parasites, particularly hook worms and whipworms. Grossly visible parasites are saved in saline for definitive parasitological identification if required. For fecal parasitological examination, the contents of the distal colon or rectum are collected, so that it is representative of the entire intestinal tract. Dark black tarry contents (Fig. 8.6) is indicative of bleeding, and a thorough search for a source of blood including upper respiratory or gastrointestinal tract bleeding from mucosal erosion and ulceration should be sought.

Figure 8.7 Small intestine of an adult dog. Approximate size of a transverse section opened along the anti-mesenteric border for appropriate fixation.

Sections of intestine are taken for fixation (Fig. 8.7) and loops can be tied off with plastic zip ties or strings to prevent spillage of intestinal contents for ancillary testing (bacteriology, virology, parasitology) (Fig. 8.8). A minimum of six sections are routinely taken from the gastrointestinal tract in the dog and the cat (see Appendix 3 and Fig. 18.1). These include sections of the fundic and pyloric mucosa of the stomach, and sections of the duodenum, jejunum, ileocecal junction, and colon. Additional sections of jejunum, rectum and any lesions can also be taken. When sampling a large discrete lesion (ulcer, abscess, mass), sections should be taken at the junction between grossly normal and abnormal tissues to assess the degree of local invasion. If a neoplastic process is suspected, the regional lymph nodes should be examined carefully and sampled for histology whether gross lesions are found or not. For histology, approximately 3 cm segments of intestine are transected and opened along the anti-mesenteric border using forceps and blunt-tipped scissors (Fig. 8.7). Segments of intestine

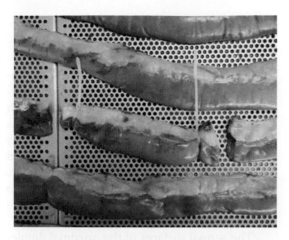

Figure 8.8 Small intestine of an adult dog with a loop tied with plastic zip ties for ancillary testing.

should never be dropped directly in fixative without completely opening each end so that the mucosa is exposed to the fixative immediately after collection. Placing unopened intestinal segments in fixative delays fixation and causes significant histological artifacts. Once histological sections have been taken, the remaining intestinal tract can be linearized, if this has not already been done, to facilitate complete examination of the lumen and mucosa. Incise the mesentery from the intestine along the mesenteric attachment. Then, a small incision is made through the wall, and extended in either direction with blunt-tipped scissors.

The wall of the stomach and intestine is evaluated for changes in color, appearance and thickness. The location and distribution of changes are recorded according to the location along the intestinal tract and the length of bowel affected, and in relation to the specific layers that are involved; mucosa, submucosa, muscularis, and serosa. The appearance of the mucosa is first assessed without washing or handling (squeezing, pinching, rubbing, or scrapping). Besides postmortem decomposition contributing to significant artifacts, handling of the gastrointestinal mucosa can significantly compromise the accuracy of histological assessment. Because Peyer's patches throughout the small intestine

often display histological changes indicative of subclinical viral infection or bacterial colonization, they should be sampled routinely. Once sampling for histology is completed, the remaining tract can be washed gently with running water and examined more closely for the presence of mucosal lesions.

The large intestine normally contains a variable amount of pasty, dark green to brown contents. Abnormally firm to hard fecal material might indicate constipation, obstipation or impaction. When hard fecal material is found in conjunction with a distended and thin-walled bowel, megacolon should be suspected. Hard fecal balls should be broken up and evaluated for the presence of foreign material such as bone fragments or sand. Finally, the mesenteric and colic lymph nodes are examined and sections are routinely fixed for histological examination.

8.4   Special Techniques

If the history or initial examination are indicative of oral or dental disease, these structures can be examined more thoroughly by sectioning the right and left vertical ramus of the mandible with an oscillating saw behind the last mandibular molar teeth #411–311 in the dog and #409–309 in the cat. After removing the jaw by gentle dissection of the surrounding skeletal muscles, the oral structures are examined more closely. The maxillary structures including the hard palate can be removed for further examination by making a transverse section behind the last maxillary molar teeth #110–210 in the dog and #109–209 in the cat. If necessary, the maxilla can be cut in half by making a sagittal section through the midline of the hard palate using a vibrating saw. Similarly, the mandible can be cut at the intermandibular symphysis. The mandible and maxilla are placed in fixative for at least 24 hours before complete decalcification and sectioning for histology.

Fresh segments of stomach or small intestine can be mounted in a petri dish filled with water and the mucosa or serosa examined under a dissecting microscope to further assess the presence of serosal or mucosal changes including damage, vascular, or lymphatic alterations.

The surface mucosa of the small and large intestine and any nodule or mass can be further assessed by making touch impression smears on glass slides. At least three or more slides should be prepared for each sample in order to allow for more than one staining method to be made and accommodate for potential breakage or loss of slides during processing. These slides can be stained with the Wright Giemsa stain for cytological assessment of exfoliated cells or search for parasitic eggs, coccidia, or cryptosporidia particularly in young dogs and cats from kennels or shelters. Detection of bacteria including acid fast organisms can be done by staining with Gram stain and Ziehl–Nielsen, or Fite Faraco, respectively. Intestinal contents can be collected for negative staining and detection of viruses by transmission electron microscopy.

If detailed histological examination of the stomach or intestine is critical, individual sections are pinned flat, serosa down, on a piece of pre-labelled, thick cardboard, or dental wax before immersion in fixative. Note that longer segments are needed since the pinned ends will be damaged and no longer usable. The flattened pieces of tissue are easier to orient during the embedding procedure and allow a more complete histological assessment particularly when the villous length to crypt depth ratio needs to be determined more accurately. For scanning or transmission electron microscopy, the contents in individual segments should be rinsed out of the lumen with buffered neutral saline prior to fixation.

8.5 Common Artifacts and Postmortem Changes

1) The fundic mucosa of the stomach can sometimes be diffusely dark red to pink from normal physiological hyperemia associated with digestion and should not be interpreted as hemorrhage. Gastric hemorrhages are usually slightly raised, darker red to black, and extend within the mucosa and submucosa on section. Histological examination should be pursued to provide a more definitive assessment when the significance of this gross change is uncertain.

2) The serosal surfaces of the proximal duodenum and pylorus of the stomach can have locally extensive green to yellow orange areas of discoloration associated with postmortem imbibition of bile acid through the gall bladder wall.

3) The presence of a small amount of creamy white mucoid material on the mucosal surface of the stomach and intestine is normal and represents sloughed epithelial cells admixed with debris and mucus.

4) A common postmortem change is distention of the stomach and intestine with gas and black to green discoloration of the wall caused by bacterial fermentation of the gut contents.

5) A common postmortem artifact in the large intestinal mucosa and sometimes the gastric mucosa is multiple longitudinal dark red to black linear streaks (tiger stripes; Fig. 8.9). These are caused by postmortem contraction of the smooth muscles and pooling of blood within the mucosal blood vessels. They can be red to black depending on the postmortem interval and degree of red blood cell lysis by bacteria and production of iron sulfide.

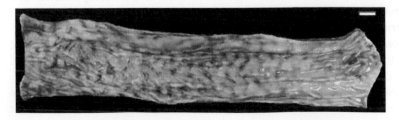

Figure 8.9 Opened colon from a young adult dog with moderate postmortem autolysis resulting in prominent longitudinal dark red to black linear streaks (tiger stripe artifact) on the mucosal surface.

6) The intestinal mucosa autolyzes very rapidly after death and the intestinal epithelium will slough into the lumen and leave denuded villi on histological examination when the postmortem interval is greater than 48 hours and the carcass is kept at room temperature without adequate refrigeration.

7) Individual segments of intestine can telescope into more distal segments resulting in postmortem intussusception. Unlike antemortem intussusception, which is difficult to reduce, postmortem intussusception is easily reducible and lacks the characteristic segmental swelling, redness and sometimes necrosis of the intestinal wall seen with an antemortem lesion.

Bibliography

Anderson, KL. N.d. Ultrasonography of the GI tract, CVM 6105 (online publication: www academic-server.cvm.umn.edu/radiology/CVM6105/2011/Anderson/pdf/USofGI.pdf, accessed August 11, 2016).

Dellmann, HD, Brown, EM. 1993. *Textbook of Veterinary Histology*, 4th edn, pp. 205–264. Philadelphia, PA: Lea & Febiger.

Floyd MR. 1991. The modified Triadan system: nomenclature for veterinary dentistry. *J Vet Dent* 8(4):18–19.

9

The Liver and Pancreas

9.1 Anatomy Review

9.1.1 The Liver

The liver is the largest gland in the body, representing 3–4% of total body weight in adult dogs and cats and up to 6% in puppies and kittens. Changes in liver weight are a sensitive indicator of hepatotoxicity, help support a diagnosis of hepatic hypertrophy or atrophy, reflect perturbations in metabolism, and correlate well with histopathologic changes. Normally, the liver lies completely under the rib cage and the cranial face is molded to the surface of the diaphragm (see Fig. 3.24).

The caudal, or visceral surface, lies in contact with the stomach, duodenum, pancreas, and right kidney, all of which but the pancreas produce impressions (Fig. 9.1). The left side of the liver, consisting of medial and lateral lobes, extends caudally to the 10th intercostal space. The quadrate lobe lies in a fissure that separates the right medial and left medial liver lobes and is variably fused to the right medial lobe. The right side of the liver is also divided into medial and lateral lobes and extends to the 12th (last) intercostal space. The caudate lobe has a caudate process, a papillary process and an isthmus that joins them. The isthmus lies between the posterior vena cava dorsally and the portal vein ventrally. The caudolateral portion of the caudate process is deeply recessed by the cranial pole of the right kidney. The papillary process extends to the left and forward from its attachment

to the caudate lobe, lies in the lesser curvature of the stomach and is loosely enveloped by the lesser omentum. The liver lobes are fused near the central porta hepatis but the degree of fusion varies between animals (Fig. 9.2).

The left and right lateral liver lobes are attached to the diaphragm by the triangular ligaments. The left medial, quadrate and right medial liver lobes are attached to the diaphragm by the coronary ligaments, which are formed by folds of the serous and fibrous coats that cover the liver. The falciform ligament, a remnant of the umbilical vein derived from the ventral mesentery, extends caudally from the liver and diaphragm to the umbilicus. In adults the falciform ligament is filled with fat. The hepatorenal ligament is variable in occurrence but when present extends from the medial aspect of the renal fossa in the caudate process to the ventral surface of the right kidney.

The portal vein (Fig. 9.3) is formed by the confluence of the cranial and caudal mesenteric veins and the gastrosplenic vein. It originates in the root of the mesojejunum and runs cranially with the hepatic artery to form part of the ventral boundary of the epiploic foramen. The common hepatic artery arises from the celiac artery and branches into 3–5 proper hepatic arteries that enter the hilus of the liver. When three proper hepatic arteries are present, the right branch arises first and supplies the right lateral and caudate liver lobes. The middle branch perfuses the dorsal aspect of the quadrate

Necropsy Guide for Dogs, Cats, and Small Mammals, First Edition. Edited by Sean P. McDonough and Teresa Southard.
© 2017 John Wiley & Sons, Inc. Published 2017 by John Wiley & Sons, Inc.
Companion Website: www.wiley.com/go/mcdonough/necropsy

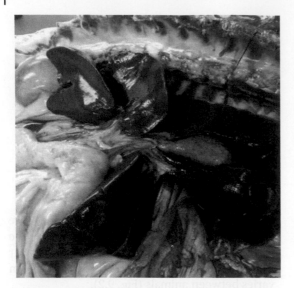

Figure 9.1 The visceral surface of the liver is in contact with the stomach, duodenum, pancreas, and right kidney.

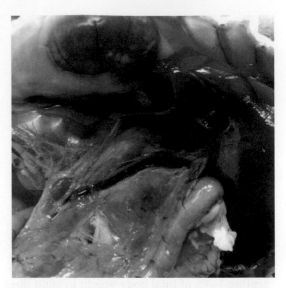

Figure 9.3 The portal vein arises in the mesojejunum and passes over the angle of the pancreas before entering the liver.

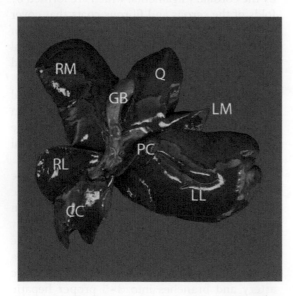

Figure 9.2 The liver consists of six lobes: Left lateral (LL), left medial (LM), quadrate (Q), right medial (RM), right lateral (RL), and caudate lobes. The caudate lobe has a caudate process (CC) and a papillary process (PC). The gall bladder (GB) lies between the quadrate and right medial liver lobes and the adventitia of the body and neck is fused with Glisson's capsule of the liver.

lobe and the right medial liver lobe. The left branch supplies the left lateral lobe and parts of the left medial and quadrate lobes. Before the left proper hepatic artery enters the hilus, it gives rise to the cystic artery that supplies the gall bladder.

The gall bladder is an ovate vesicle that lies between the quadrate and right medial liver lobes (Fig. 9.2). In cats, the gall bladder is occasionally bilobed (Fig. 9.4). The cranial, rounded, blind end of the gall bladder is referred to as the fundus, the large middle portion is the body and the slender, tapering extremity is the neck. The cystic duct extends from the neck of the gall bladder to the junction with the first bile duct tributary from the liver. From here the excretory channel becomes known as the common bile duct (Fig. 9.5). The distal end of the common bile duct enters the duodenum obliquely and forms a low, longitudinal ridge that represents the intramural course. The bile duct terminates on a small mound of tissue at the end of the ridge termed the major duodenal papilla (Fig. 9.6). To one side is the slit-like opening of the minor pancreatic bile duct.

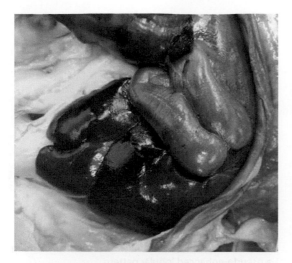

Figure 9.4 A bilobed gall bladder is a relatively common incidental finding in a cat.

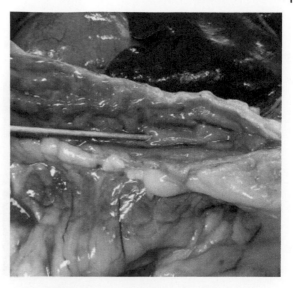

Figure 9.6 The intramural bile duct terminates at the major duodenal papilla (ampulla of Vater). The probe passes through the sphincter of Oddi, which is a muscular valve that controls the flow of bile and pancreatic secretions into the duodenum.

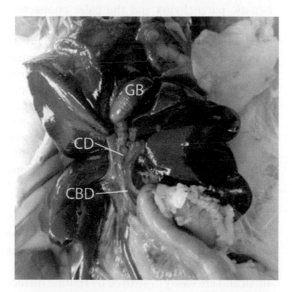

Figure 9.5 The cystic duct (CD) extends from the neck of the gall bladder (GB) to the junction with the first bile duct tributary from the liver. From here it is referred to as the common bile duct (CBD).

9.1.2 The Pancreas

Islet, acinar, and ductal cells of the pancreas all develop from dual outpouchings of the developing duodenum. The dorsal pancreatic diverticulum forms the left lobe of the pancreas. The ventral diverticulum arises as a secondary branch of the hepatic diverticulum and forms the right lobe. The acinar cells arise as diverticula from the sides of the smaller terminal branches of the developing ducts. Rotation of the dorsal and ventral diverticula results in partial fusion of the pancreatic lobes.

The pancreas is a pink-grey, coarsely lobulated organ with two elongated lobes that are fused at the head or pancreatic angle. The portal vein crosses the pancreatic angle where the two lobes are joined (Fig. 9.3). The right lobe is long, thin, and runs in the mesoduodenum next to the descending duodenum. The left lobe lies in the dorsal sheet of the greater omentum and is only about two-thirds as long but is up to 1.5 times wider than the right (Fig. 9.7). The lobules create a somewhat nodular surface with irregularly rounded projections along the margins. The Islets of Langerhans, not visible grossly, are microendocrine organs surrounded by exocrine tissue. Islets are randomly distributed throughout the pancreas, but in the dog are most plentiful in the left limb.

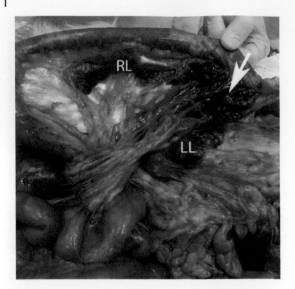

Figure 9.7 The right lobe (RL) of the pancreas runs parallel to descending duodenum while the left lobe (LL) lies in the dorsal sheet of the greater omentum. The arrow points to an area of postmortem autolytic leakage of blood in the pancreas. Autolysis releases lysosomal enzymes that disrupt blood vessels, leading to accumulation of blood in the pancreatic parenchyma.

In almost all cases, the pancreas has two ducts for transporting its exocrine secretion, reflecting the dual origins of the gland. The accessory pancreatic duct is the major excretory pathway in the dog and enters the duodenum at the minor papilla. The pancreatic duct opens onto the major duodenal papilla and is the only duct in the majority of cats. Variations in the pattern of the ducts are common in dogs. About 75% of dogs have two ducts. A few dogs have only an accessory duct while others have three openings into the duodenum. Within the pancreas, the duct systems fuse to form an anastomotic network.

9.2 *In Situ* Evaluation and Removal

9.2.1 The Liver

The normal liver is uniformly dark red-brown, smooth, and firm but friable. Careful inspection reveals a diffuse, finely mottled appearance due

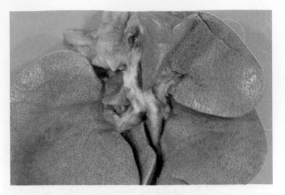

Figure 9.8 Enhanced lobular (reticular) pattern in the liver. Care should be taken not to over interpret this finding at necropsy as autolysis, especially in the cat, will unmask the stromal framework of the liver creating a pseudo-enhanced lobular pattern.

to the contrast in color between the darker hepatic parenchyma and the paler connective tissue that outlines the hepatic lobules, which are approximately 1 mm in diameter. Diffuse pallor may indicate an intracellular accumulation such as lipid (e.g., feline hepatic lipidosis syndrome) or glycogen (e.g., "steroid hepatopathy"). Cholestasis frequently imparts a green tinge to the parenchyma. An enhanced lobular pattern may be due to a variety of processes including zonal hepatic lipidosis (e.g., hepatoxicity, early Feline Hepatic Lipidosis Syndrome, cholangitis/cholangiohepatitis, leukemia, and lymphoma; Fig. 9.8).

Before disturbing the viscera, the abdomen should be carefully explored for congenital or acquired extrahepatic portosystemic shunts (PSS). Acquired portosystemic shunts may be small and are easily destroyed by routine dissection so they must be identified before removal of the viscera. Thin-walled, tortuous vessels occur most often in the mesenteric veins, right renal vein, or gonadal vein. Precaval acquired portosystemic shunts, which are most common in people and cause esophageal varices, are rare in dogs and cats. Most congenital shunts run near the epiploic foramen. To locate the epiploic foramen, fan out the mesentery of the descending loop of the duodenum by retracting this segment of intestine ventrally and to the left,

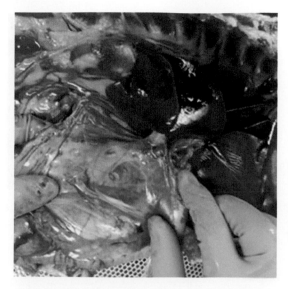

Figure 9.9 Most congenital extrahepatic portocaval shunts run near the epiploic foramen. Spread out the mesentery by retracting the duodenum ventrally. The epiploic foramen is bounded by the portal vein ventrally and the caudal vena cava dorsally.

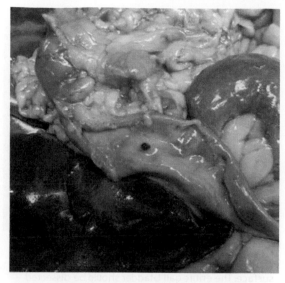

Figure 9.10 Assess the patency of the extrahepatic biliary tree by manual compression of the gall bladder. A short incision through the antimesenteric border of the descending duodenum to visualize the greater duodenal papilla can facilitate evaluation. Note the bead of bile forming at the sphincter of Oddi.

exposing the right kidney, portal vein and caudal vena cava (Fig. 9.9). The ventral border is formed by the portal vein while the caudal vena cava is the dorsal border. It may be necessary to expose the celiac artery in order to visualize a PSS terminating on the caudal vena cava. Portoazygos shunts often penetrate the diaphragm at the level of the crura or aortic hiatus. The azygos and hemiazygos veins and the aorta travel through the aortic hiatus and the caudal vena cava passes through the caval foramen. Any other vessel of significant size (portal or splenic vein in size) that penetrates the diaphragm is likely to be a portoazygos shunt. If a left, central or right divisional intrahepatic shunt is suspected, trace the intrahepatic portal vein.

Assess the size and course of the cystic and common bile ducts and inspect the gall bladder for size, color and thickness of the wall. The cystic artery ramifies primarily on the surface of the gall bladder attached to the liver and is best evaluated by histopathology. Patency of the extrahepatic biliary tree is assessed by manual

compression of the gall bladder. A short incision through the antimesenteric border of the descending duodenum to visualize the greater duodenal papilla can facilitate evaluation (Fig. 9.10). Aerobic and anaerobic cultures of an aseptic aspirate of bile and a sample of gall bladder wall are indicated if bacterial infection is suspected. Bacteria most often are within or adhered to biliary sludge and cytologic smears of this material offer the greatest chance of detection. The gall bladder can be opened now or after removal of the liver (Fig. 9.11). Note the volume and character of the bile. Normal bile is thin, clear, and green-tinged with a mucoid texture. The volume of the gall bladder in normal dogs (fasted 12 h) is typically <1 ml/kg (median 0.6 ml/kg; range 0.4–1.9 ml/kg). Anorexia often leads to gall bladder distention (lack of food-induced cholecystokinin release from the duodenal mucosa) and the accumulation of soft, green-black bilirubinate sludge due to bile concentration as a consequence of water resorption. For these reasons it is imperative that the

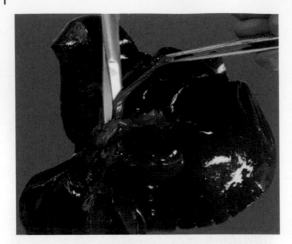

Figure 9.11 The gall bladder is opened to inspect the character of the content and examine the mucosal surface. The entire gall bladder should be dissected away from its attachments to the quadrate and right medial liver lobes.

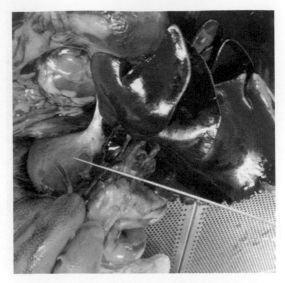

Figure 9.12 The hepatoduodenal ligament can be incised to separate the liver from the rest of the alimentary tract.

volume and character of bile only be interpreted in light of histopathological evaluation of the gall bladder and liver.

The liver can be removed with the gastrointestinal tract. Alternatively, after the adrenal glands have been collected and the pluck removed, cut the root of the mesentery and incise the hepatoduodenal ligament, taking care to keep the pancreas with the small intestine (Fig. 9.12). The stomach and intestines with the pancreas are harvested as a single unit. Next, sever the diaphragm from its attachments to the lumbar vertebrae, left costal arch, and the sternum and lift the liver and attached diaphragm out of the abdomen. At this point, it is easy to cut the diaphragm away from the liver and spread it out for detailed examination (See Fig. 7.4).

9.2.2 The Pancreas

The location, size, shape, color, consistency, and texture of the pancreas are assessed during gross inspection of the rest of the abdominal viscera. The pancreas accounts for approximately 0.25% of total body weight, but weighing the pancreas is seldom indicated. It is most

convenient to open the proximal duodenum to identify the major and minor papillae and trace the pancreatic and accessory ducts prior to removal. Special attention should be given to assessing the peripancreatic fat. Saponification of peripancreatic fat from pancreatitis forms pearly white, gritty foci (Fig. 9.13). The common bile duct should be carefully evaluated in cases of pancreatitis since inflammation centered on the pancreas can extend to involve the common bile duct. The pancreas will remain associated with the stomach and descending duodenum when the gastrointestinal tract is removed.

9.3 Organ Examination, Sectioning, and Fixation

9.3.1 The Liver

The gall bladder mucosa autolyzes rapidly due to the effects of bile and it is best to sample the gall bladder first. Incise the gall bladder from the fundus to the neck and inspect the mucosal lining as well as a cross section of the wall (Fig. 9.11). If the cystic and common bile ducts

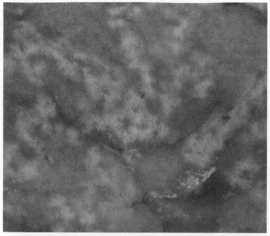

Figure 9.13 Peripancreatic fat necrosis. Pancreatitis can release digestive enzymes into adjacent tissues causing fat necrosis. Necrotic fat can form pearly white, mineralized, gritty foci (saponification).

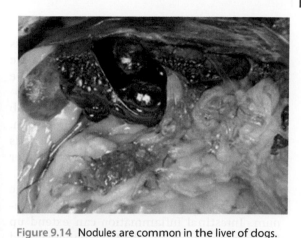

Figure 9.14 Nodules are common in the liver of dogs. Older dogs almost invariably have foci of nodular hyperplasia. Metastatic neoplasia is common in the liver while hepatocellular carcinomas, which resemble hepatic parenchyma, are fairly rare.

are large enough, open their lumens longitudinally with a small pair of blunt-end scissors. Alternatively, transverse slices perpendicular to the course of the extrahepatic bile ducts every 1–2 cm will allow for inspection of the wall and lumen.

Each lobe of the liver should be inspected for size, shape, and color and palpated for texture and consistency. Inspection slices should be made every 2 cm and the cut surface examined. Representative sections should be collected from at least two or three lobes along with any lesions. If portal vein hypoperfusion is suspected, be sure to collect sections from lobes other than the caudate, since changes may be less obvious in the caudate liver lobe because it is perfused by the first branch from the hepatic artery.

Hepatic nodules in an otherwise normal liver from middle-aged and older dogs most likely represent nodular hyperplasia. Rinsing a slice of liver in formalin can accentuate these nodules. In contrast, regenerative nodules represent compensatory hyperplasia and arise from a background of hepatic injury, atrophy and fibrosis. Metastatic neoplasia is common in the liver and if a mass lesion is found, a diligent search for a primary should be undertaken. Hepatocellular carcinoma is relatively rare (0.5% of all canine tumors). The tumors may present as a single large mass, multiple smaller masses in multiple lobes or disseminated throughout the liver. They typically resemble hepatic parenchyma (Fig. 9.14). Biliary cystadenomas and cholangiocellular carcinomas are most common in cats.

If hepatic lipid accumulation is severe, the liver will be enlarged, pale yellow with a greasy texture and a friable consistency (Fig. 9.15). Floating a section of liver in water or formalin can confirm severe hepatic lipidosis but is unreliable in mild to moderate cases. If hepatic lipidosis is suspected, sections should be collected in formalin with a request for special stains for lipids. Tissue processing leeches out lipids and their presence can only be demonstrated with special stains (e.g., Oil Red O) on frozen sections of either fresh or formalin-fixed tissue. Animals with hepatic amyloidosis most often present with hemoabdomen due to liver fracture. Amyloid can be detected by first painting the cut surface with an iodine solution and then rinsing in dilute sulfuric acid, which will turn amyloid from brown to purple.

9.3.2 The Pancreas

Make inspection slices every 1–2 cm across the short axis of both limbs. In the cat, chronic pancreatitis is more common in the left lobe so both lobes should be examined histopathologically. Collect a section of the right limb with a cross section of attached duodenum. A longitudinal section of the left limb aids recognition when blocking in the tissues after fixation.

In the cat, the hepatic duct fuses with the pancreatic duct prior to entering the duodenum. Intestinal inflammation can extend up the common duct to affect the pancreas and liver ("triaditis"). The large Pacinian corpuscles of the cat pancreas appear as pinpoint white foci in the interlobular trabeculae. Rarely, these laminated pressure receptors can be as large as 1–3 mm. Nodular hyperplasia of the exocrine pancreas is common in older dogs and cats without evidence of prior pancreatic injury. Foci of nodular hyperplasia are scattered throughout the pancreas as grey-white, firm, smooth nodules of variable size (Fig. 9.16).

9.4 Common Artifacts and Postmortem Changes

9.4.1 The Liver

1) Imbibition of bile quickly stains the hepatic parenchyma adjacent to the gall bladder and extrahepatic bile ducts dark green-black (see Fig. 2.10A). Imbibition of bile will also stain the duodenum around the greater duodenal papilla.

2) Pseudomelanosis, grey to black areas of discoloration, develops where the liver is in contact with the intestine (Fig. 9.17). Iron released from degraded hemoglobin combines with hydrogen sulfide produced by bacteria in the gut lumen to produce iron sulfide (FeS).

3) Moderate autolysis often unmasks the reticular framework of the liver, creating a pseudo-enhanced reticular pattern, especially in cats.

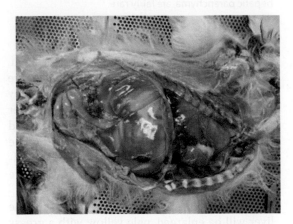

Figure 9.15 Hepatic lipidosis in a recently weaned puppy. The liver is diffusely pale yellow, greasy and has a friable consistency.

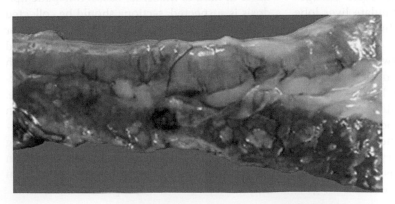

Figure 9.16 Pancreatic nodular hyperplasia is a common, incidental finding in old dogs and, less often, in cats.

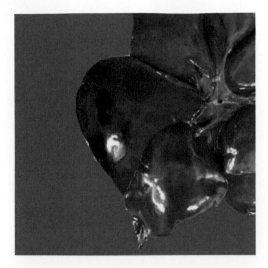

Figure 9.17 Pseudomelanosis. Loops of intestine in contact with the liver during the postmortem period will discolor the surface grey to black. Iron released from degraded hemoglobin combines with hydrogen sulfide produced by bacteria in the gut lumen to produce iron sulfide (FeS), a visible black precipitate.

4) Translocation of anaerobic saprophytes can generate irregular pale foci and gas bubbles in the parenchyma. In advanced cases of autolysis, the liver will be soft, pasty and grey-brown.

9.4.2 The Pancreas

1) The pancreas autolyzes rapidly. Initially, the normal pink-grey color changes to a dark red-brown and then green as autolysis becomes advanced.
2) Postmortem hemorrhage into the pancreatic interstitium due to autodigestion by pancreatic enzymes is common in dogs but seen less often in cats (Fig. 9.7). This must not be misinterpreted as necrohemorrhagic pancreatitis. If in doubt, submit a section for histopathologic confirmation.

Bibliography

Bindhu, M, Yano, B, Sellers, RS, Perry, R, Morton D, Roome, N, Johnson JK, Schafer K. 2007. Evaluation of organ weights for rodent and non-rodent toxicity studies: a review of regulatory guidelines and a survey of current practices. *Toxicol Pathol* 35:742–750.

De Cock, HEV, Forman, MA, Farver TB, Marks SL. 2007. Prevalence of histopathologic characteristics of pancreatitis in cats. *Vet Pathol* 44:39–49.

Eichhorn, EP, Boyden, EA. 1955. The choledochoduodenal junction in the dog; a restudy of Oddi's sphincter. *Am J Anat* 97:431–451.

Evans HE and deLahunta A. 2013. Liver. In: *Miller's Anatomy of the Dog*. 4th edn. St. Louis, MO: Elsevier Saunders; pp. 327–333

Ramstedt, KL, Center, SA, Randolph, JF, Yeager, AE, Erb, HN, Warner, KL. 2008. Changes in gall bladder volume in healthy dogs after food was withheld for 12 hours followed by ingestion of a meal or a meal containing erythromycin. *Am J Vet Res* 69:647–651.

Weiss, DJ, Gagne, JM, Armstrong, PJ.1996. Relationship between inflammatory hepatic disease and inflammatory bowel disease, pancreatitis, and nephritis in cats. *J Am Vet Med Assoc* 209(6):1114–1116.

10

The Urogenital System

10.1 Anatomy Review

The urogenital system is composed of two geographically and embryologically related, but functionally diverse, tracts: the reproductive tract and the urinary tract. These tracts are considered together because they converge distally and are often removed together (Fig 10.1).

The urinary tract consists of the kidneys, ureters, urinary bladder, and urethra. The kidneys are located against the sublumbar muscles, under the peritoneum. The left kidney is more caudal than the right, with the left at the level of the second to fourth vertebral bodies and the right at the level of the first to third. Cat kidneys are characterized by prominent capsular veins, while the surface of dog kidneys is smooth. Cat kidneys are also lighter in color than dog kidneys, due to increased lipid content of the tubular epithelial cells. (Fig. 10.2) The blood supply to the kidneys is the renal artery, usually the fifth branch off of the abdominal aorta (after the unpaired celiac artery and cranial mesenteric artery and the paired adrenal arteries). The renal veins drain directly into the caudal vena cava. The adrenal glands are located medial to the kidneys and cranial to the renal vessels.

The ureters run along the psoas muscle before entering the bladder. In males, the ureters cross the ductus deferens prior to connecting with the bladder. The ureters continue a short distance within the smooth muscle of the bladder before opening into the lumen. The bladder varies greatly in size and the wall varies in thickness, depending on the degree of distension by urine.

The components of the reproductive tract vary depending on the species, sex, and whether the animal has been neutered. For intact females, the tract consists of ovaries, oviducts, uterine horns and body, cervix, vagina, and vulva, while spayed females have only the uterine stump, cervix, vagina, and vulva. Intact male reproductive tracts include testes, epididymides, ductus (or vas) deferens, and accessory sex glands (prostate in dogs; prostate and bulbourethral glands in cats). In neutered males, the testes and epididymides are absent.

The ovaries are located at the caudal poles of the kidneys, at the level of the third (right) or fourth (left) lumbar vertebral bodies. They are ovoid and flattened and often encased in adipose tissue. In spayed animals, the remnant of the ovarian pedicle and possibly suture material can usually be found at this location. The uterus consists of a very short body with two horns that extend from the level of the aortic bifurcation to the caudal aspect of the ovary. In spayed animals, only the uterine stump and ligated uterine vessels (in larger animals) will be present. The short oviduct is a coiled tube that runs beside the ovary. The cervix is not apparent from an external view of the reproductive tract, but can be palpated as a thick band of smooth muscle at the junction between the uterine body and the vagina. The vestibule is the distal part of the female reproductive tract, extending from the external urethr. The external urethral orifice opens into the vestibule on the ventral aspect.

Necropsy Guide for Dogs, Cats, and Small Mammals, First Edition. Edited by Sean P. McDonough and Teresa Southard.
© 2017 John Wiley & Sons, Inc. Published 2017 by John Wiley & Sons, Inc.
Companion Website: www.wiley.com/go/mcdonough/necropsy

(A)

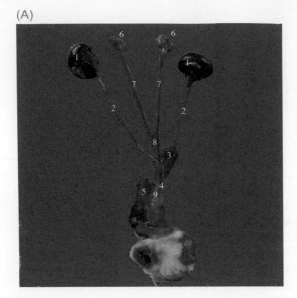

(B)

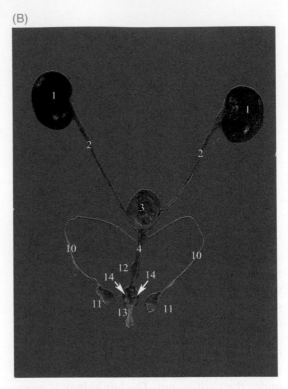

Figure 10.1 Anatomy of the urogenital tract of a female dog (10.1A) and a male cat (10.1B). Structures are labeled as follows: 1. Kidney; 2. Ureter; 3. Bladder; 4. Urethra; 5. Rectum; 6. Ovary; 7. Uterine horns; 8. Uterine body; 9. Vagina; 10. Ductus (vas) deferens; 11. Testis and epididymis; 12. Prostate gland; 13. Penile urethra; 14. Bulbourethral glands.

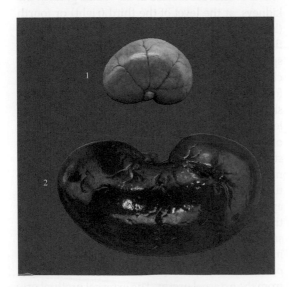

Figure 10.2 Cat and dog kidneys. The cat kidney (1) is lighter in color, due to increased fat content, and has prominent subcapsular veins, compared to dog kidney (2).

In males, the testes usually descend into the scrotum by 2–4 months of age. In younger animals or cryptorchid animals, the testes may be located anywhere from the caudal aspect of the kidney to the inguinal canal. In dogs, testes are oriented horizontally while feline testes have a more vertical position. In both species, testes are ovoid and flattened laterally with the epididymis along the dorsal aspect. The ductus deferens is continuous with the tail of the epididymis and travels, along with the testicular vessels, in the spermatic cord to the internal inguinal ring. In dogs, but not in cats, the ductus widens into an ampulla prior to joining the urethra. The prostate gland is located at the base of the bladder, cranial to the junction between the urethra and ductus deferens. In the dog, the prostate gland surrounds the urethra. In cats, the gland is more "U" shaped, leaving the ventral aspect of the urethra uncovered. At the base of the penis, the urethra becomes ensheathed in the urethralis muscle. The canine penis lies between the thighs, with the prepuce and urethral opening near the level of the umbilicus. The feline penis is shorter and oriented caudoventrally. The glans is covered by keratinized papilla that develop in the first few months after birth and regress following castration.

10.2 *In Situ* Evaluation and Removal

The sex of the animal and the external genitalia are evaluated during the external examination. Scrotal testes are palpated and removed while reflecting the skin from the abdominal cavity. Removal is very similar to castration, by incising the skin and opening the tunica vaginalis to expose the testes, epididymis, and spermatic cord. If the testes are removed and set aside for later examination, it is helpful to leave a longer section of spermatic cord attached to the left testis to allow for differentiation. If no scrotal testes are found in a reportedly intact animal, the search can continue once the abdomen is open.

After opening the abdominal cavity and before any organs are removed, the kidneys should be located and counted (there should be two), the status of the female reproductive tract (intact or spayed) should be assessed, and the inguinal canal and abdomen can be searched for missing testes. This search is facilitated by locating the ductus deferens and following it cranially to the kidney or caudally to the inguinal canal. The remainder of the *in situ* examination is best accomplished after the other abdominal organs (gastrointestinal tract, liver, spleen, and pancreas) have been removed (Fig. 10.3). It is a good idea to mark the right kidney with a small transverse cut into the parenchyma, so that the left and right kidneys can be differentiated once removed from the body. Also, if there is urine in the bladder, a sample of urine can be collected with a needle and syringe (see Fig. 3.40).

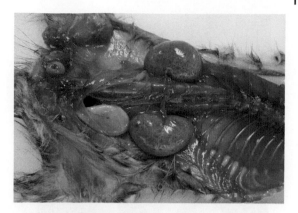

Figure 10.3 The feline urinary tract *in situ* after removal of the thoracic viscera, intestine, liver and spleen. This kitten's kidneys are enlarged and contain hundreds of fluid filled cysts (polycystic kidney disease).

The kidneys, ureters, bladder, urethra, female reproductive tract (if present), prostate (in males) can be removed as a unit by cutting the renal vessels and reflecting the tract caudally. Depending on the particular case, the distal tract can be either severed, by pulling the tract caudally and cutting the urethra and vagina within the pelvic cavity, or the pelvis can be split and the entire tract removed. The pelvis can be split either by cutting the pubis and ischium on both sides of the pubic symphysis or by cutting these bones on the right side and cutting the ileum (Fig. 10.4). Use a knife or scalpel to cut the soft tissue around the perineum and remove the distal part of the rectum, along with the vagina, vestibule, urethra, and anus.

10.3 Organ Examination, Sectioning, and Fixation

10.3.1 Kidneys

The size of the left and right kidneys should be compared for evidence of atrophy or hypertrophy. Variation in size is best documented by weighing the organs once all the perirenal adipose tissue has been removed. In adult animals, the kidneys should approximately 0.4% of the body weight (see Appendix 1). In young animals

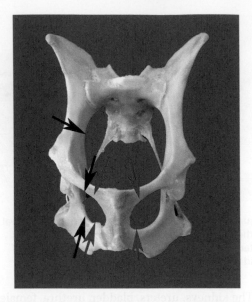

Figure 10.4 The pelvis can be split by two methods. The pubis and ischium can be cut on both sides of the pubic symphysis (red arrows) or the pubis and ischium can be cut on the right side of the symphysis and the body of the right ilium cut (black arrows). The section of bone is removed so that the distal urethra, vagina and rectum can be extracted with the rest of the genitourinary tract.

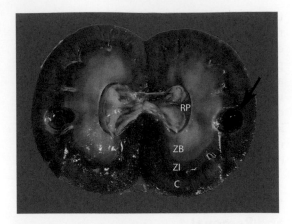

Figure 10.5 Examination of the cut surface of the kidney. The cortex (C) is brown, and the medulla is divided into two parts: The outer zona intermedia (ZI) is red, while the inner zonal basalis (ZB) is white to grey with radiating striations. The corticomedullary junction should be distinct and the renal pelvis (RP) should be slit-like. This kidney has a focal cyst at the corticomedullary junction (arrow).

(less than 6 months) the percentage of body weight should be closer to 1%. Evaluation of the surface of the kidneys requires removal of the capsule. This is easiest to do after sectioning the kidneys. Longitudinal sectioning of the kidneys allows optimal evaluation of the parenchyma and renal pelvis. Once the kidneys are sectioned, the capsule should be removed and the capsular surface inspected, followed by examination of the cut surface of the kidney (Fig. 10.5). The demarcation between the medulla and cortex should be sharp, although it may undulate slightly at the level of the arcuate arteries. The cortex is red-brown and, in a fresh cadaver, the glomeruli are visible as regularly spaced, 1 mm diameter nodules. The medulla is divided into two parts. The external part, the zona intermedia, is dark red. The inner part, the zona basalis, is greyish red with radial striations. The renal pelvis should be a slit-like space between the renal medulla and the adipose tissue and vessels

at the hilus. Collecting a transverse section of the right kidney and a longitudinal section of the left kidney allows differentiation between the two for histopathology (Fig. 10.6).

10.3.2 Ureters

Ureters should be examined for evidence of dilation, obstruction, inflammation, or stenosis. Initial examination of the diameter of the ureter can be deceiving, since this structure is often surrounded by a layer of adipose tissue. The diameter and patency of the lumen is best assessed by opening the ureter using small, blunt-ended scissors.

10.3.3 Bladder and Urethra

Open the lumen of the bladder and urethra along the ventral aspect using blunt-tipped scissors. Start by making an incision into the apex of the bladder and then extend the incision caudally. In cats and small dogs, the entire bladder and urethra can be fixed in formalin. In large dogs, collect a thin strip of the urinary bladder, from apex to trigone (Fig. 10.7). Urethra is typically collected only if abnormalities are suspected.

Figure 10.6 Histology samples from the kidney. A transverse section is collected from the right kidney (1) and a longitudinal section from the left kidney (2).

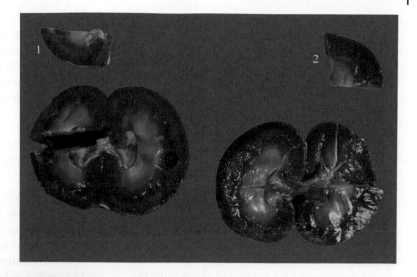

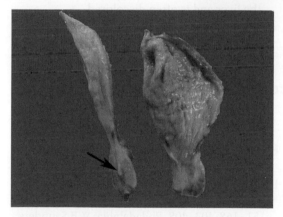

Figure 10.7 Histology sample from the bladder. A longitudinal strip of bladder, including apex, body, trigone and proximal urethra is collected. This section includes the ureteral orifice (arrow).

10.3.4 Ovaries

Compare the size of the left and right ovaries. There may be some variation in size due to the presence of follicles and corpora lutea at different stages of development. For large dogs, section the left ovary longitudinally and the right ovary transversely for fixation. In cats and small dogs, the entire female reproductive tract can be submitted for histopathology.

10.3.5 Oviduct/Uterus/Cervix/Vagina

Open the lumen of both uterine horns using blunt scissors and continue the incision caudally and through the cervix into the vagina. Note the color, consistency, and odor of any fluid in the lumen. If the animal is pregnant, note the sex and crown to rump length of all fetuses (see Chapter 16, Table 16.1).

10.3.6 Testes/Epididymides/Ductus Deferens

Compare the size of the left and right testis and epididymis. In large dogs, section the left testis and epididymis longitudinally and the right testis and epididymis transversely for examination and fixation. Testes from large dogs can be serially sectioned to look for masses or areas of inflammation. For small dogs and cats, the testes and epididymides can be submitted together. The ductus deferens can be examined in the spermatic cord attached to the testes and also where they enter the bladder. These structures are not sampled as part of a routine necropsy, but any lesions should be collected.

10.3.7 Prostate Gland

In cats and small dogs, the prostate gland is collected and fixed with the bladder and urethra.

In large dogs, the gland may be large enough to serially section to look for masses or evidence of inflammation.

10.3.8 Bulbourethral Gland (Cats Only)

These small glands lie on either side of the urethra at the base of the penis (Fig. 10.1). While it is valuable to know the location of these glands, collection and examination of them is not part of a routine necropsy.

10.3.9 Distal Colon/Rectum/Anus

Although not part of the urogenital system, the distal part of the gastrointestinal tract is removed with the urinary and reproductive organs and should be examined along with the other pelvic organs. Open the distal colon using scissors and collect a section for histopathology. The anal sacs are located on either side of the distal rectum, and care should be taken not to rupture these glands during removal of the tract. Sections of the anal sacs should be collected if there is evidence of a mass, hemorrhage, or necrosis.

10.4 Special Techniques

If urinary obstruction is expected, care should be taken to remove the entire urinary tract to the distal urethral orifice. The ureters, bladder and urethra should be opened and inspected for evidence of blockage.

Urinary calculi can be collected and submitted for identification. Some diagnostic laboratories provide this service free of charge.

If renal amyloidosis is suspected, the cut surface of the kidney can be soaked in Lugol's Iodine solution and then rinsed in sulfuric acid. Amyloid in the glomeruli (more common in dogs) or interstitium (more common in cats) will stain black.

Touch imprints of the cut surface of the kidney can reveal calcium oxalate crystals. With an appropriate history, this finding is diagnostic for ethylene glycol toxicity.

A refractometer or urine dipstick can be used to test urine collected from the bladder.

10.5 Common Artifacts and Postmortem Changes

1) Kidneys autolyze rapidly and the parenchyma can be very soft if the postmortem interval is prolonged.
2) White streaks in the renal cortex are normal in well-conditioned animals.
3) The cranial pole of the right kidney is against the liver and is often discolored.
4) The down side kidney will be darker and may ooze blood when sectioned (livor mortis).
5) The urine in autolyzed carcasses can appear cloudy due to sloughing of urothelial cells
6) A segmental area of the urethra is often dark red (postmortem congestion).

Bibliography

Dyce KM, Sack WO, Wensing CJG. 1996. *Textbook of Veterinary Anatomy*, 2nd edn, pp. 151–168, 403–408. Philadelphia: WB Saunders Company.

Evans HE, de Lahunta A. 2012. *Miller's Anatomy of the Dog*, 4th edn. New York: Elsevier, electronic edition.

King JM, Roth-Johnson L, Newson, ME. 2007. *The Necropsy Book: A Guide for Veterinary Students, Residents, Clinicians, Pathologists, and Biological Researchers*. 5th edn. Gurnee, Ill.: Charles Louis Davis, DVM Foundation.

Maxie, M Grant. 2015. In *Jubb, Kennedy and Palmer's Pathology of Domestic Animals*, Vol. 2, 6th edn. New York: Saunders Elsevier.

11

The Nervous System

11.1   Anatomy Review

Initially during embryologic development, as the neural tube is developing, three rudimentary brain regions develop: the prosencephalon, the mesencephalon, and the rhombencephalon. As development proceeds, the prosencephalon develops two distinct regions: the telencephalon and diencephalon, while the rhombencephalon develops into the metencephalon and the myelencephalon. These divisions are important to understand in the greater anatomic organization of the brain. The telencephalon is composed of the two cerebral hemispheres and associated lateral ventricles while the diencephalon includes the thalamus, hypothalamus, and third ventricle as it passes both dorsally and ventrally through the thalamus. The mesencephalon is traversed dorso-centrally by the mesencephalic aqueduct which carries cerebrospinal fluid from the lateral ventricles to the fourth ventricles and eventually to the lateral aperture. The metencephalon gives rise to the pons along the ventral portion and the cerebellum dorsally. Lastly the myelencephalon becomes the medulla oblongata. The spinal cord develops from a spherical tube to its mature form characterized by a prominent dorsal medial sulcus and ventral median fissure with laterally arranged white matter and a central, "butterfly" of grey matter. The central canal runs the middle of the spinal cord and carries cerebrospinal fluid. A basic understanding of the development of the brain is especially helpful as it relates to malformations commonly encountered in the central nervous system.

Nervous tissue is a dynamic structure, studded with numerous cell types. While a full discussion of the functions of these cell types is outside the scope of this text, a brief review is provided here for context. Neurons populate the grey matter of the brain and spinal cord and their axons traverse both the grey and white matter where they are surrounded by myelin. In the central nervous system, myelin is produced by oligodendrocytes which are found in both the grey and white matter, in the latter forming chains of cells. Astrocytes provide a myriad of functions in the brain including helping form the blood-brain barrier as well as various physiologic roles. Microglia are the resident macrophages of the central nervous system and have phagocytic behavior as well as a variety of other immunologic roles. Blood vessels are scattered throughout the parenchyma. Specialized cells line the ventricles (ependyma) and aid in production and flow of cerebrospinal fluid. Epithelial cells line the choroid plexus with an additional role in the production of cerebrospinal fluid.

As the neural tube is forming, a population of cells that has its origin in neuroepithelium coalesces dorsal to the developing tube. This collection of cells, referred to as the neural crest, is the origin of the neurons and the Schwann cells of the peripheral nervous system. These neural crest cells migrate away from the dorsal midline and form ganglia of the sympathetic

Necropsy Guide for Dogs, Cats, and Small Mammals, First Edition. Edited by Sean P. McDonough and Teresa Southard.
© 2017 John Wiley & Sons, Inc. Published 2017 by John Wiley & Sons, Inc.
Companion Website: www.wiley.com/go/mcdonough/necropsy

trunk, dorsal root, enteric plexi, and parasympathetic ganglia. Once at these locations, these cells provide the hubs for synaptic transmission throughout the body.

11.2   *In Situ* Evaluation and Removal

11.2.1   Brain

Access to the brain and spinal cord can be difficult without the proper tools. To remove the brain and spinal cord, a knife/scalpel and saw (a vibrating saw works best; however, a standard bone saw is also acceptable) is required. Remove the head as described in Chapter 3. Once the head is removed from the cervical spine, the foramen magnum can be evaluated for coning of the cerebellum (indicating increased intracranial pressure) or malformative abnormalities of the occipital bone (Fig. 11.1). To facilitate removal of the brain from the calvaria, it is important to remove as much muscle and soft tissue as possible including the large temporalis muscle and the soft tissue attachments around the caudal occipital bone (Fig. 11.2).

Once the soft tissue is removed, locate the zygomatic process of the frontal bone. The initial cut is made transversally through the frontal bone at the level of this process (Fig. 11.2). The other two cuts run from the edge of the transverse cut to the medial aspect of the occipital condyle at the foramen magnum on both the left and the right side. This will produce three cuts in the bone. If the cuts have been made to completion, a T tool can be directed into the transverse cut and the bone flap can be lifted towards the prosector (Fig. 11.3). As the bone is removed, the dura will pull away from the brain and the tentorium cerebelli will also be removed. If the tentorium remains *in situ*, it can be carefully dissected away from the brain. Depending on the force with which the dura pulls away from the brain, it may bring along with it the pineal gland (normally nestled between the occipital lobes and

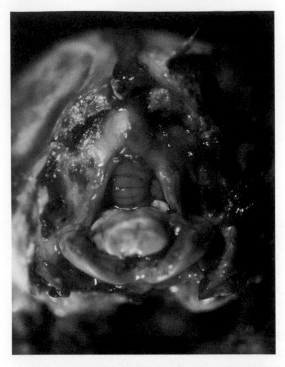

Figure 11.1 Canine skull, caudal aspect. The occipital bone is malformed with a wedge-shaped section of occipital bone absent exposing the subjacent cerebellar vermis.

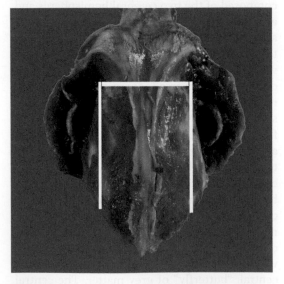

Figure 11.2 Canine skull. To remove the calvaria, the skeletal muscle is cleaned from the skull. Three cuts are made: two cuts along either side of the occipital condyle connecting to a transverse cut in the frontal bone, just caudal to the orbit.

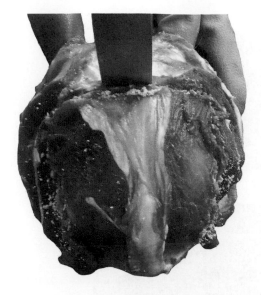

Figure 11.3 Canine skull. A T tool is used to remove the calvarial bone.

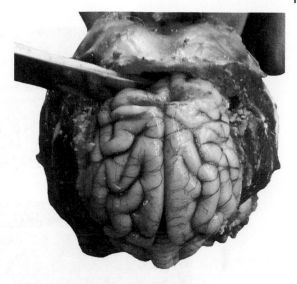

Figure 11.4 Canine skull. To remove the brain following detachment of the olfactory bulbs and ventral nerve attachments, a scalpel handle can be used to draw the brain out of the calvaria with the assistance of gravity.

dorsal to the mesencephalon) and the choroid plexi from the lateral ventricle. Neither of these structures should be confused with a neoplasm.

At this point, the prosector is ready to remove the brain. Resting the skull upright on the ramus of the mandible, the olfactory peduncles can be cut as well as the ventral attachments of the cranial nerves. Visualization of the cranial nerve attachments may be facilitated by flipping the skull 180° and allowing gravity to pull the brain towards the prosector, thereby better exposing the cranial nerves. Once these attachments are cut, the skull can be tilted to allow gravity to help draw the brain out of the calvaria (Fig. 11.4). Any other remaining soft tissue attachments can be cut at this time. Careful examination of the cranial nerves as they pass through their associated foramina should be made at this time.

In neonatal animals the skull bones are not fused or ossified, so it is much easier to use bone cutting forceps to cut the bone away and expose the brain. Use of a saw in neonatal and small mammals increases the risk of inadvertent postmortem damage to the brain.

11.2.2 Spinal Cord

Removal of the spinal cord can be a particular challenge. Prior to removal of the spinal cord, as much muscle and soft tissue as possible must be removed from around the vertebrae. For cats, small bone forceps can be used to remove the dorsal aspect of the vertebrae; however, this is very difficult to do in a dog, especially larger breeds. An oscillating saw is the best option for getting the spinal cord out of the spinal canal. Using the saw, cuts are made at approximately 45° off dorsal midline so that when the dorsal part of the vertebrae are removed the cord can be visualized *in situ* (Fig. 11.5A). The bone of the atlas and axis is typically quite dense and therefore can be difficult to cut into. Once the prosector feels the saw blade drop into the vertebral column, the saw must be backed out. It is relatively easy to inadvertently traumatize the spinal cord with the saw. Once the entire dorsal portions of all vertebrae have been removed down to the terminus of the spinal cord (cauda equina), the cord can be removed (Fig. 11.5B). Grasping the dura around the first cervical spinal cord column with forceps and pulling upward, a scalpel

(A)

(B)

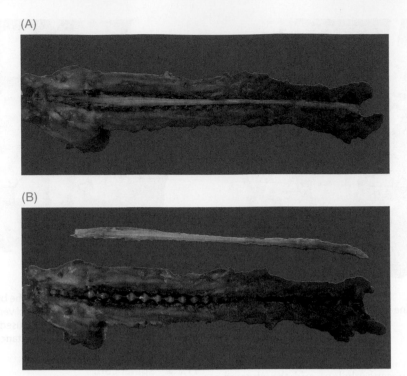

Figure 11.5 Canine vertebral column. Bilateral cuts are made through the dorsal laminae of the vertebrae at approximately 45° off midline, and the bone removed to expose the spinal cord (A). The dura is grasped with forceps and the spinal nerve roots cut to extract the spinal cord (B).

blade can be used to cut the nerve roots as they exit the spinal cord. Applying enough pressure to pull the cord towards you, but not so much as to rip the cord, it will allow for the dorsal root ganglia to be visualized and the nerve can be cut distal to the ganglia so that the ganglia are included to the complete dissection. Once fixed, a transverse and longitudinal section of cord should be examined from each section of spinal cord (i.e., cervical, thoracic, lumbar, and sacral).

11.2.3 Peripheral Nerves

If the clinical history suggests a focal or diffuse peripheral nervous system disorder, examination of the peripheral nerves is of utmost importance. The cranial nerves are best visualized when the brain is removed (Fig. 11.6B) and if a specific nerve is believed to be implicated (i.e., facial neuritis), then the nerve can be dissected from its origin and followed to the tissues that it innervates.

Other nerves can be selected based on clinical history. To sample a generic peripheral nerve during the complete necropsy, the sciatic nerve is the most accessible. The sciatic nerve passes over the greater ischiatic notch of the ischium and then eventually passes caudal to the femur on the lateral surface of the adductor muscle. Dissection deep to the semimembranosus, semitendinosus, and biceps femoris will reveal the large nerve contained within the deep fascia (see Fig. 3.13).

11.3 Organ Examination, Sectioning, and Fixation

11.3.1 Brain

The surface of the brain (Fig. 11.6A) should be examined for any defects or imperfections related to an extraparenchymal neoplasm. Examination of the gyri for either complete absence (lissencephaly),

(A)

(B)

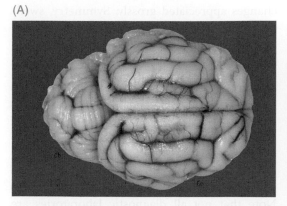

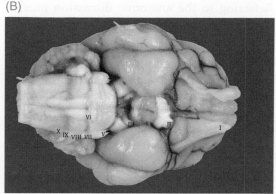

Figure 11.6 Feline brain, dorsal and ventral aspects. (A) Normal feline brain illustrating normal cerebral (Ce) to cerebellar size (Cb). (B) Ventral surface of the brain with ventral brain stem and cranial nerve attachments. Attachments of cranial nerves IV and XI are not visible in this image.

increased number (polymicrogyria), or increased size (pachygyria) can be performed at this time. The meninges should be interrogated for the presence or absence of an exudate. If the presence of an exudate is suspected, touch impression smears will aid the pathologic interpretation. Symmetry of the brain should also be assessed as well as the normal arrangement of gyri and sulci, any changes in which would suggest a parenchymal lesion. Expansion of the ventricular system (hydrocephalus; Fig. 11.7) or absence of certain parts of the brain can also be performed at this time. In order to preserve the architecture of the brain, especially in small animals, the entire brain can be placed in fixative without sectioning. For small animal brains, 10% neutral-buffered formalin (NBF) is the best fixative. For larger brains, in order to facilitate uniform diffusion of fixative into the tissue, several transverse slices can be made into the brain. If electron microscopy is suggested by clinical signs and disease (i.e., storage disease), a section of brain can be placed in glutaraldehyde.

In order to dissect the brain, it is important to use a fresh, clean blade and to trim each brain the same way to achieve consistency. Before sectioning, total brain weight and cerebellar weight can be recorded. Normal cerebellar weight should be 10–12% of the total brain weight in a normal animal, with lower percentages reflecting loss of cerebellar mass (as is seen in diseases causing

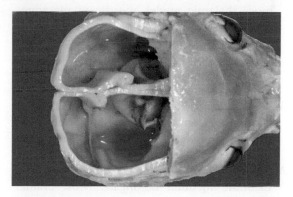

Figure 11.7 Canine, brain. Severe hydrocephalus with marked dilation of the lateral ventricles and thinning of the cerebral cortices.

loss of cerebellar cortical tissue, such as abiotrophy). One-centimeter transverse sections are made through the entire brain from the olfactory bulbs to the medulla. Once the sections are made, lay the sections in order on a cutting board from rostral to caudal. This allows for complete assessment of symmetry and color changes that may accompany a lesion. Fresh brains can sometimes mask subtle lesions, but in fixed tissue, large areas of inflammation and/or necrosis often appear dull grey and can be more easily appreciated than in the fresh specimen. It is imperative that while this dissection is proceeding, the prosector is reviewing any imaging studies that would help localize the lesion.

Referring to the anatomic discussion previously, the following systemic dissection is indicated:

Telencephalon: Rostral part of brain stem, cerebral cortices, and lateral ventricles. This allows examination of caudate nucleus, basal nuclei, and fornix.

Diencephalon: Further down the brain stem; this will allow exposure of thalamus and corpus callosum. You will see start of lateral ventricles with prominent internal capsule. Longitudinal third ventricle obvious divided into dorsal and ventral parts depending on the section examined.

Mesencephalon: This will allow exposure of more thalamic nuclei, mesencephalic aqueduct, and various parts of hippocampus depending on where slice is made. You should be able to visualize lateral and medial geniculate nuclei, which play an important role in the visual system.

Metencephalon: Remove remaining cerebrum from brain stem. This will allow visualization of pons and cerebellum. Transverse section through cerebellum.

Myelencephalon: Expansive 4th ventricle. Examine medulla oblongata. Most cranial nerves arise in the medulla, so if you are looking for a specific nucleus, this is the place to examine.

11.3.2 Spinal Cord

Similarly, the spinal cord should be left intact for complete fixation. The prosector should make note of any gross abnormalities when submitting the spinal cord especially of lesions that involve the tissues surrounding the spinal cord (i.e., bone, muscle). If the spinal cord is fixed in multiple parts, it is imperative that the different sections are labeled appropriately (i.e., the cranial portion of each section is marked with a tissue cassette).

11.3.3 Nerves

The majority of diseases that directly affect the nerves have only histologic or sub-cellular changes and therefore there are few to no changes appreciated grossly. Symmetry, swelling, and/or thinning of the nerve should be noted grossly. Examination of nerves often requires special preparation and staining procedures. Generically, a section of nerve should be affixed to a wooden tongue depressor, allowed to dry adhere to the wood, and then placed in 10% NBF. If fresh frozen sections of nerve are required for diagnostic purposes, a section of nerve can be wrapped in gauze and placed in physiologic saline. This is then shipped to the appropriate laboratory overnight on wet ice. Note that not all diagnostic laboratories are equipped to handle fresh nerve biopsies for frozen sections and therefore communication with the laboratory ahead of time is recommended.

11.4 Common Artifacts and Postmortem Changes

1) Due to the high lipid content in the brain and spinal cord, autolysis does occur at a rapid rate. Especially in neonatal and young animals this can result in nervous tissue that loses cohesion and consistency when removed from the calvaria or spinal column. Since it is difficult to maintain normal anatomy in cases like this, the brain should be immediately placed in 10% neutral buffered formalin to allow for proper fixation and minimize excess handling.

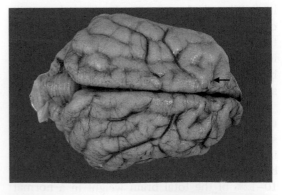

Figure 11.8 Canine, brain. The meninges in the sulci are thickened and white to tan (arrow). This is consistent with meningeal fibrosis.

Figure 11.9 Canine, spinal cord. In the spinal cord meninges are multiple plaques of dural ossification. These can contain bone marrow.

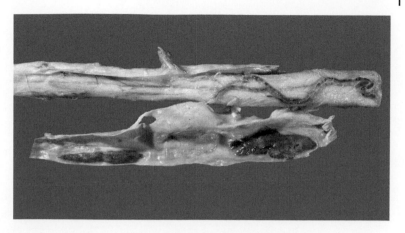

2) In addition to autolysis, if the putrefaction of brain tissue involves gas production (i.e., from bacteria), then bubbles of various sizes can develop within the parenchyma.

3) Gas bubbles can form within the meninges of the brain when the calvaria is removed. These occur due to the separation of the dura from the arachnoid which pulls the arachnoid off the pia mater and brain and allows for air to accumulate in these spaces.

4) Since removal of the brain and spinal cord requires the use of either hand-held or mechanical saws, inadvertent cutting of the parenchyma and embedding of bone fragments often occur.

5) Melanosis of the meninges is a common finding in animals that have abundant skin pigmentation like the Newfoundland dog breed.

6) Meningeal fibrosis is a common finding in aged animals. This can appear as a white to tan thickening that is most pronounced in the sulci. This is not to be confused with meningitis, which, when scraped with a knife, should peel away (Fig. 11.8).

7) A common finding in the spinal cord of middle to older aged dogs is dural ossification (formerly referred to as ossifying pachymeningitis). These regions of osseous metaplasia form in the dura and can often have their own bone marrow compartments. It is not associated with significant clinical disease and considered an incidental, age-associated finding (Fig. 11.9).

8) Congestion of the meningeal blood vessels is a common finding and typically insignificant.

Bibliography

Evans, HE, de Lahunta, A. 2012. *Miller's Anatomy of the Dog*, 4th edn. Philadelphia, PA: Elsevier Saunders.

Noden, DM, de Lahunta, A. 1985. *The Embryology of Domestic Animals: Developmental Mechanisms and Malformations*. 1st edn. Philadelphia, PA: Williams and Wilkins.

Wohlsein, P, Deschl, U, Baumgärtner, W. 2012. Nonlesions, Unusual cell types, and postmortem artifacts in the CNS of domestic animals. *Vet Pathol* 50(1):122–143.

12

The Eye and Ear

12.1 The Eye

12.1.1 Anatomy Review

The eye and the seven associated extraocular muscles reside in the orbit and are cushioned by periorbital fat. The long posterior ciliary arteries extend from the optic nerve to the equator of the globe in the horizontal plane and are an important landmark when sectioning the globe. The eyelids protect the anterior surface of the eye. They are covered with haired skin on the outer surface and the conjunctiva, a thin mucous membrane, on the inner surface. Eyelids sweep foreign material from the anterior surface of the eye and facilitate movement of tear film to the nasolacrimal drainage channels at the medial canthus. Cilia (eyelashes) are most numerous in the upper lid and are commonly lacking in the lower lid. The nictitans, or third eyelid, resides at the medial angle of the palpebral fissure and contains a flat, T-shaped piece of hyaline cartilage. The seromucoid nictitans gland is molded to the base of the cartilage. The free edge of the third eyelid may be pigmented or unpigmented.

The globe is formed by three concentric coats. The fibrous outer tunic gives the eye its shape and consists of the cornea and the sclera. The cornea is clear and refracts light. The sclera provides the site of attachment for the extraocular muscles. The sclera is separated from the cornea at the limbus. The innermost tunic is the retina. The optic nerve is an extension of the brain and is surrounded by meninges.

The thick middle vascular tunic, also referred to as the uvea, contains the choroid, ciliary body, and iris. The choroid envelopes the posterior of the globe, except at the optic nerve head, and is continuous with the ciliary body anteriorly. The tapetum is a reflective area that occupies about one-third of the superior choroid and is responsible for the eyeshine seen when a beam of light is directed into the eye. The ciliary body lies between the choroid and iris. The posterior flat portion is the pars plana and the raised anterior portion is the pars ciliaris. Zonular fibers arise from the pars ciliaris and suspend the lens behind the pupil. The ciliary body also produces aqueous humor. The iris is the most anterior portion of the uvea and is a thin, circular diaphragm with a central pupil. The anterior chamber is located between the cornea and iris and is filled with aqueous humor. Aqueous humor drains through the filtration angle at the base of the iris in the anterior chamber. The vitreous body is a gelatinous mass between the lens and the retina and helps keep the retina in place.

Ocular anatomy is complex and the reader is referred to standard reference texts for more detail (see Bibliography).

12.1.2 *In Situ* Evaluation and Removal

Antemortem ophthalmic exam findings provide the best guidance for identifying microscopic correlates. Alternatively, flattening the cornea with a glass slide and shining a penlight through

Necropsy Guide for Dogs, Cats, and Small Mammals, First Edition. Edited by Sean P. McDonough and Teresa Southard.
© 2017 John Wiley & Sons, Inc. Published 2017 by John Wiley & Sons, Inc.
Companion Website: www.wiley.com/go/mcdonough/necropsy

the pupil will illuminate intraocular structures and allow for a reasonably thorough fundic exam (Fig. 12.1). Be careful as the glass slide can erode the corneal epithelium.

Enucleation should be done gently since rough handling causes retinal detachment and artifacts in the optic nerve. Incise the skin around the globe but leave a generous margin that can be grasped with forceps for traction (see Fig. 3.45). Incise the bulbar fascia (Tenon's capsule) around the circumference of the globe near its attachment to the limbus with a scalpel blade (Fig. 12.2). Using the attached rim of haired skin for traction, sever the soft tissue anchoring the globe to the orbit, preserving as much of the optic nerve as possible (Fig. 12.3). This last step may be easier with a pair of scissors (Fig. 12.4).

Clean off the extraocular tissue and save the optic nerve for longitudinal and cross sections. Excess soft tissue delays fixative penetration, which promotes artifacts, obscures landmarks for proper orientation, and makes it harder to section the globe. Extraocular tissue can be easily removed by pinching the soft tissues between a cutting board and the necropsy knife. Keeping

the knife stationary, with the edge of the blade angled slightly away from the globe to avoid inadvertently incising it, sweep the tissues under the blade while using gentle traction (Fig. 12.5). As the tissues are cut, the globe will rotate, allowing for quick and easy removal of extraocular soft tissue. Take care not to transect the optic nerve. Leaving the optic nerve longer on the left eye will aid in distinguishing left from

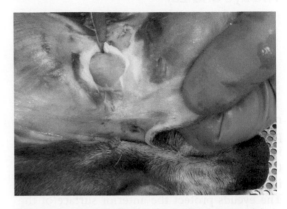

Figure 12.2 Incise the bulbar fascia (Tenon's capsule) around the circumference of the globe near its attachment to the limbus with a scalpel blade.

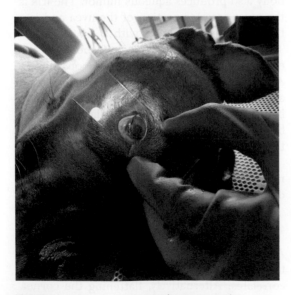

Figure 12.1 A post mortem ocular exam can be performed by carefully flattening a microscope slide against the cornea and using a penlight.

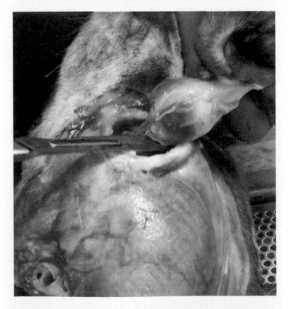

Figure 12.3 Incise the soft tissues close to the bony orbit, preserving as much of the optic nerve as possible.

Figure 12.4 Removal of the globe from the orbit may be easier with a pair of scissors rather than a scalpel blade.

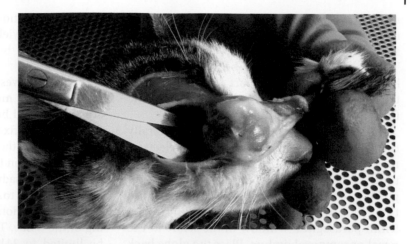

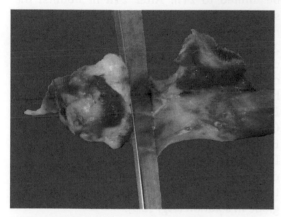

Figure 12.5 Fixation and sectioning are enhanced by removing the soft tissues from the globe. Lightly pinch the soft tissues under a knife blade, with the edge angled slightly away from the globe. Keeping the knife steady, sweep the tissues under the knife edge while applying traction.

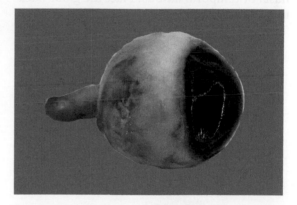

Figure 12.6 A globe freed of soft tissues, suitable for immersion fixation. Leaving the optic nerve longer on the left eye aids in distinguishing the left and right globes.

right (Fig. 12.6). Alternatively, a spot of dye, typically applied to the superior aspect of the globe, can be used to distinguish right from left as well as maintain orientation (Fig. 12.7).

12.1.3 Examination, Sectioning, and Fixation

Once the globe has been removed, transillumination with a bright light projected through the cornea can help identify shadows of intraocular masses. All fixatives and fixation techniques will create at least some degree of artifact. Small

animal eyes typically fix in 24 h but large globes should be fixed for 48 h before sectioning. Likewise, globes with masses and those filled with exudate or blood require longer fixation. It is generally not advisable to open the eye or to cut windows into the sclera.

Fixation by immersion is the most common technique and generally yields good results. Immersion in 10 times the volume of fixative as quickly as possible after death helps to minimize autolysis. Wrapping the eye in several layers of gauze can help ensure 360° fixation. Injecting fixative into the vitreous body can help the vitreous body fix as an intact gel, which reduces sectioning artifact. Use a small gauge needle (25–27 ga) and a small volume of fixative (e.g., 0.15–0.3 ml). Insert the needle through the sclera parallel to the long posterior ciliary artery. The point of entry should be posterior to the limbus and at the widest part of the globe so as to avoid the lens (Fig. 12.8). Slowly inject the fixative until the globe feels turgid.

Cutting windows into the globe is generally restricted to research cases and for electron microscopy. Never cut windows into a globe until it has been hardened first. Place the globe in 6% glutaraldehyde for 1–2 h. Position the globe with the cornea down and cut a 5 mm parasagittal window in the sclera at the nasal or temporal limbus. Place the globe back in 6% paraformaldehyde to complete fixation.

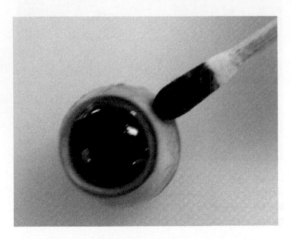

Figure 12.7 A dot of dye on one globe can be used to distinguish left from right and can also help with orientation. A spot of india ink is being applied to the sclera at the superior aspect of the right eye.

Perfusion fixation is generally not recommended as it yields inconsistent results and creates spaces beneath the retinal pigment epithelium.

Several fixatives are commonly employed to fix globes. The most commonly used fixatives are 10% neutral buffered formalin and Bouin's fluid. Formalin fixation is generally adequate for routine histopathology but Bouin's fluid yields better results and is preferred for enucleated globes. The disadvantages to Bouin's fluid are that it is highly toxic, potentially explosive, and prolonged fixation results in excessive hardening of the tissue. Thus, fixation in Bouin's must be limited to 24 h. After 24 h in Bouin's, the samples are rinsed in cold tap water until no more yellow color washes out (approximately 2–3 min). Once the globe has been trimmed, the cassettes are placed in a properly labeled container of 70% ethanol and submitted to the histology laboratory. An excellent alternative to Bouin's fluid is Davidson's fixative (Table 12.1). Cellular preservation is nearly as good as with Bouin's fluid but is considerably less toxic. Davidson's fixative and Bouin's fluid cause the cornea to turn white (opaque) so gross examination should be performed before placing the globe in solution (Fig. 12.9).

For all mammals except primates, the standard section is taken from the vertical, mid-sagittal plane of the globe. Place the cornea down and identify the optic nerve and long posterior ciliary artery. Position the blade next to the optic nerve and perpendicular to the long posterior ciliary artery. Using a sharp 130 mm trimming

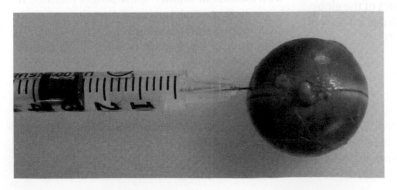

Figure 12.8 Injecting a small volume of fixative (0.15–0.3 ml) into the vitreous body can reduce sectioning artifacts. The injection is made parallel to the long posterior ciliary artery caudal to the lens until the globe is turgid.

Table 12.1 Davidson's Fixative for Eyes*.

95% ethyl alcohol	30 ml
10% neutral buffered formalin	20 ml
Glacial acetic acid	10 ml
Distilled water	30 ml

* Any desired volume can be made using the formula above. The globe must be removed from the fixative after 24 h. Rinse the tissue under running water (2–3 min) and then transfer into 10% neutral buffered formalin. The globe can now be sectioned and processed normally.

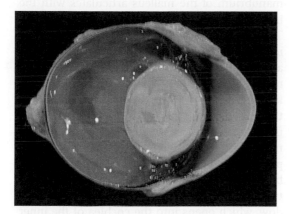

Figure 12.9 Bouin's fluid provides excellent preservation but causes the cornea to become opaque so gross examination should be performed before immersing the globe in fixative. Excellent quality photographs can be achieved by placing the calotte on a pedestal of modeling clay in a black bowl and just barely submerging the surface of the specimen in water.

blade, make one smooth, downward, and forward cut until you meet resistance from the lens. Grasp each end of the blade firmly and push straight down through the lens and cornea. Complete the cut by pulling back on the blade to yield two calottes.

Inspect both calottes for gross changes and take photographs. Excellent photographs can be achieved by positioning the globe on a pedestal of modeling clay in a small black bowl and just barely submerging the cut surface in water (Fig. 12.9). After taking photographs, make a second cut parallel to the first but avoid the lens. This second cut can be facilitated by placing the

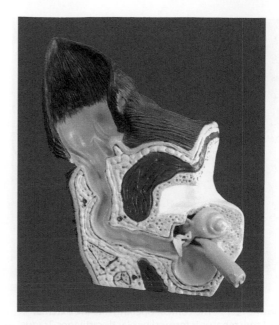

Figure 12.10 A model showing the external, middle and inner portions of the ear.

calotte cut-edge down in a deep megacassette and running the blade along the edge of the cassette, slicing off any tissue that is too tall. Be sure the calotte is not compressed when the lid is closed.

12.2 The Ear

12.2.1 Anatomy Review

The ear is divided into three parts: the external ear, the middle ear, and the inner ear (Fig. 12.10). The external ear consists of the pinna (ear flap) and the external auditory meatus. The auricular cartilage forms the pinna and most of the ear canal. The shape of the pinna in dogs is characteristic of the breed and may be erect, semi-erect, or pendulant. Pinnae in cats are erect or folded (Scottish fold cats). A complex group of skeletal muscles, all innervated by the facial nerve, control pinnal movements. Haired skin covers the convex and concave surfaces of the pinnae.

The conical opening into the external auditory meatus is formed by elastic cartilages that include the tragus, antitragus, helix, antihelix,

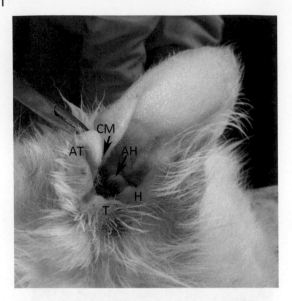

Figure 12.11 The conical opening into the external auditory meatus is formed by elastic cartilages. Tragus (T); Antitragus (AT); Cutaneous marginal pouch (CM); Antihelix (AH); and Helix (H).

and the marginal pouch (Fig. 12.11). This conical opening gradually narrows into the vertical ear canal that runs ventrally and slightly rostrally. The vertical canal bends medially and continues as the horizontal ear canal. The horizontal ear canal is surrounded by and merges into the osseous acoustic meatus near the skull. Hair follicle numbers within the external ear canal decrease toward the tympanic membrane. In dogs, ceruminous glands, specialized apocrine glands, become more numerous near the tympanic membrane while the density of sebaceous glands is greatest near the external acoustic meatus.

The tympanic membrane separates the external and middle ears. The external surface of the tympanic membrane is covered by a thin layer of squamous epithelium that overlies a thin stromal layer. The dorsal part is termed the pars flaccida and is relatively flaccid and very vascular. The large pars tensa is located ventrally and is normally translucent.

The middle ear is filled with air and contains the tympanic bulla, the medial face of the tympanic

membrane, the auditory ossicles with their associated muscles and ligaments and the auditory tube. The auditory tube communicates with the nasopharynx and equalizes pressure on either side of the tympanic membrane. The opening of the auditory tube lies in the rostral-medial portion at the middle level of the middle ear. The auditory ossicles are three small bones that transmit air vibration from the tympanic membrane to the inner ear. The anterior, or long, process of the malleus is embedded in the middle of the dorsal portion of the pars tensa. The caudal manubrium of the malleus articulates with the incus, which in turn articulates with the stapes. The stapes covers the oval (vestibular) window into the inner ear and is fused to the cartilage along the rim of the opening. In the dog, the manubrium is C-shaped with the concave surface facing cranially. In cats the manubrium is relatively larger and straighter. The tensor tympani muscle attaches to the malleus and draws it medially, tensing the tympanic membrane. The promontory of the pertrosal part of the temporal bone lies opposite the mid-dorsal portion of the tympanic membrane. The oval (cochlear) window, which opens into the cochlea of the inner ear, lies at the caudal end of the promontory.

The ventral tympanic bulla is the largest portion of the middle ear (Fig. 12.12). The septum bulla is a ridge of bone that projects from the medial wall of the tympanic bulla. The free edge of the septum bulla in dogs often has numerous small bony ossicles giving it a roughened texture (Fig. 12.13). The septum bulla in cats is very large and divides the tympanic bulla into a large ventromedial part and a smaller dorsolateral portion.

The inner ear is an osseous labyrinth within the petrous temporal bone and consists of the cochlea, semicircular canals, and vestibule. The bony labyrinth is separated from a slightly smaller inner membranous labyrinth. The membranous labyrinth is filled with potassium-rich endolymph. The space between the outer surface of the membranous labyrinth and the osseous labyrinth is filled with perilymph that is continuous with the cerebral spinal fluid through the perilymphatic duct. No communication exists between the endolymphatic and perilymphatic spaces.

The osseous cochlea is a hollow spiral of bone in the promontory of the petrous temporal bone that turns around a central axis termed the modiolus. The blind apex is the cupula. The cochlea contains three ducts; a lower tympanic duct, an upper vestibular duct, and a medial cochlear duct. The tympanic and vestibular ducts are filled with perilymph. The cochlear duct is filled with endolymph and contains the Organ of Corti that transduces auditory signals into nerve impulses. A fibrous basilar membrane forms the floor of the cochlear duct and separates the endolymph from the perilymph of the tympanic duct. The thin vestibular membrane forms the roof of the cochlear duct and separates it from the vestibular duct.

The vestibule is an irregular oval space filled with perilymph in the medial part of the petrous temporal bone continuous with the scala tympani and contains the utricle and the saccule. The utricle is an elliptical recess in the caudodorsal medial wall while the saccule is a spherical recess anteroventral to the utricle. The macules are small areas of the lining epithelium in the utricle and saccule that contain hair cells with multiple stereocilia and a single kinocilium. The kinocilium is embedded in a gelatinous membrane loaded with calcium carbonate protein granules known as otoliths. Movement of the gelatinous membrane stimulates the hair cells. The utricle and saccule both detect linear acceleration while the saccule also detects head tilt.

The oval window, covered by the base of the stapes, resides in the lateral wall of the vestibule. The round window is ventral to the oval window. Movement of the tympanic membrane causes the stapes to move inwards, compressing the fluid in the cochlea. This leads to outward movement of the membrane covering the round window allowing the perilymph to move within the cochlea. Vibrations in the perilymph are transmitted to the endolymph. The result is stimulation of the hair cells in the Organ of Corti, located on the basilar membrane of the cochlear duct, and transduction of sound.

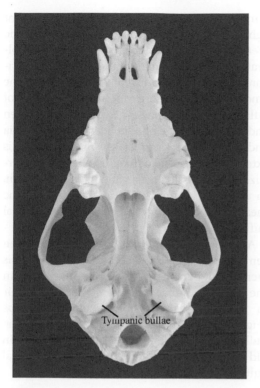

Figure 12.12 The tympanic bullae are hollow, hemispherical expansions of the temporal bone on the ventral aspect of the skull.

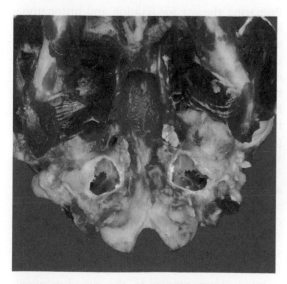

Figure 12.13 A view of the opened tympanic bullae. The free edge of the septum bulla in dogs often has numerous small bony ossicles giving it a roughened texture.

The semicircular canals open into the vestibule caudally. Each canal forms approximately two-thirds of a circle and they are oriented perpendicular to one another. The membranous ducts in the semicircular canals are filled with endolymph while the osseous canals contain perilymph. Each canal has two crura that communicate with the vestibules. Near the junction with the vestibule, each canal has one crus that is dilated into an ampulla. Within the ampulla is the crista ampularis, a cone-shaped collection of hair cells that is covered by a gelatinous membrane and detects angular acceleration (rotation).

12.2.2 *In Situ* Evaluation and Removal

Evaluation of the ear at necropsy is often limited to the pinna and the opening to the external ear canal. However, thorough assessment of the ear requires careful examination of the middle and inner portions of the ear as well.

Transect the cartilage of the external auditory meatus as close as possible to the osseous external meatus (Fig. 12.14). This is most convenient when reflecting the skin from the skull in preparation to

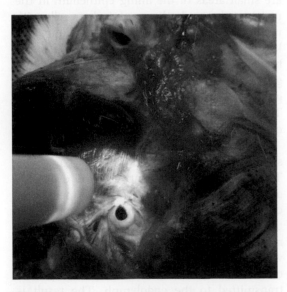

Figure 12.14 Examination of the tympanic membrane for perforation, discoloration or thickening is best done after removing the external ear as close to the bony external acoustic meatus as possible.

remove the brain. Use an otoscope or a bright light and a magnifying lens to assess the tympanic membrane for perforation, thickening or discoloration. Incise the length of the vertical and horizontal ear canals and examine the lining for the amount and appearance of cerumen, signs of inflammation and masses. Cytology of cerumen and exudates is helpful in identifying bacteria and/or yeast. In cases of severe chronic otitis externa, the cartilage of the ear canal may mineralize or even ossify, necessitating decalcification. In this case, submit the entire external acoustic meatus to the histology laboratory in 10% neutral buffered formalin.

After the brain and pituitary gland have been removed, turn the skull so the ventral aspect is facing you. Scrape the musculature away from the tympanic bullae and open them with a pair of sharp, pointed bone cutting forceps (Fig. 12.13). Normally the bone of the tympanic bulla is thin but bilateral thickening is normal in old tomcats. Swabs should be taken for bacterial culture if any fluid or exudate is present.

12.2.3 Examination, Sectioning, and Fixation

Preparing the ear for fixation and histopathological examination requires care and strict attention to landmarks. Saw transversely through the base of the skull on a line that extends between the caudal edge of the zygomatic arches and through the middle of the hypophyseal fossa (Fig. 12.15). The middle and inner ears will be contained within the caudal portion of the skull. At this point, place the specimen in 10% neutral buffered formalin.

Once the specimen that contains the middle and inner ears is fixed (minimum of 48 h), the specimen must be decalcified. Normally, decalcification takes 2 weeks for cat ears and 3 weeks for the ear from a medium-sized dog. Using a sharp razor blade, cut along a line that extends from the inner third of the occipital condyle to a point 1–2 mm medial to the round window opposite where the auricular cartilage articulates with the bony opening of the external acoustic

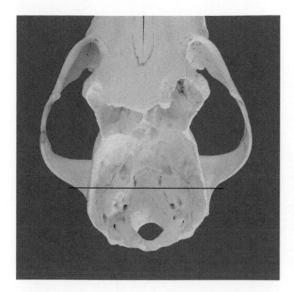

Figure 12.15 Landmarks for isolating the middle and inner ears for decalcification and histopathological evaluation. Saw transversely through the base of the skull on a line that extends between the caudal edge of the zygomatic arches and through the middle of the hypophyseal fossa. The middle and inner ears will be contained within the caudal aspect of the skull.

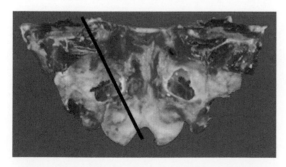

Figure 12.16 Landmarks for sectioning the middle and inner ears for histopathological evaluation. Cut along a line that extends from the inner third of the occipital condyle to a point 1–2 mm medial to the round window (note: a fresh specimen is used to better illustrate the relevant anatomy but it is better to fix and decalcify the specimen before sectioning.

meatus (Fig. 12.16). The resulting section will include the tympanic bulla, the vestibule, the cochlea of the inner ear, and a narrow portion of

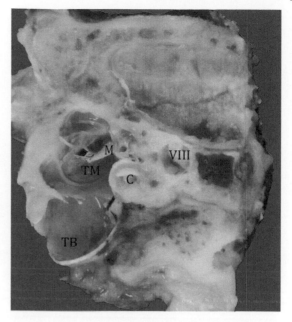

Figure 12.17 A section through the promontory of the petrous temporal bone showing the tympanic bulla (TB), the vestibule (V), the cochlea (C), the vestibulocochlear nerve (VIII) and the tympanic membrane (TM) and manubrium of the malleus (M). (Note: the perforation in the tympanic membrane is an artifact.)

the external ear canal with the tympanic membrane and manubrium of the malleus (Fig. 12.17).

Bibliography

Griffin, CE. 2009. Otitis: Anatomy that every practitioner should know. *Compend Vet Med* Nov. 504–521.

Njaa, BL, Sula, MJM. 2012. Collection and preparation of dog and cat ears for histologic examination. *Vet Clin N Am: SA* 42(6):1127–1135.

Murphy, CJ, Polock RVS. 1993. The eye. In: *Miller's Anatomy of the Dog*, 3rd edn. HE Evans (ed.), Philadelphia, PA: WB Saunders.

Sameulson, DA. 2007. Ophthalmic Anatomy. In: *Veterinary Ophthalmology*, 4th edn. KN Gelatt (ed.), Ames, IA: Blackwell Publishing.

13

The Endocrine System

13.1 Anatomy Review

13.1.1 The Pituitary Gland

The pituitary gland (hypophysis) is situated at the base of the brain caudal to the optic chiasm, between the piriform areas and anterior to the mammillary bodies. The gland consists of the adenohypophysis and the neurohypophysis connected to the overlying hypothalamus by the infundibular stalk. It rests in the hypophyseal fossa formed by the basisphenoid bone (see Figs. 3.46 and 5.1D). The neurohypophysis is derived from a down growth of diencephalic neuroectoderm while the adenohypophysis comes from a dorsal evagination of oropharyngeal ectoderm called the craniopharyngeal duct (Rathke's pouch). The pars intermedia forms where these two structures come in contact. The developing basisphenoid bone eventually separates the craniopharyngeal duct from the oropharynx. The rest of the cells in Rathke's pouch proliferate to form the pars distalis, the largest part of the adenohypophysis, which surrounds the developing pars intermedia and pars nervosa. As the pars nervosa enlarges, it collapses the lumen of Rathke's pouch resulting in a residual lumen called Rathke's cleft. A dorsal projection of cells along the infundibular stalk forms the pars tuberalis, which serves as a scaffold for the hypophyseal portal system as it courses from the median eminence to the pars distalis.

13.1.2 The Thyroid and Parathyroid Glands

The thyroid is a single gland with two lateral lobes that lie on either side of the trachea in dogs and cats. A thin isthmus of thyroid tissue extending across the ventral aspect of the trachea joins the caudal poles of the two lobes in some dogs, seen most common in brachycephalic breeds. The cranial pole of the right lobe lies opposite the caudal edge of the cricoid cartilage or the first tracheal ring (Fig. 13.1). The left lobe usually is situated 1–3 cartilage rings caudal to the right. Grossly, the thyroid lobes are flattened and ellipsoid with the dorsal surface wider than the ventral surface. The caudal poles are small and often pointed while the cranial poles are wider and rounded. The two lobes are more or less symmetrical and extend along the trachea for 5–6 tracheal rings. On external and cut surfaces the lobes are uniformly dark red-brown.

The parathyroid glands are intimately associated with the thyroid gland but they are distinct in function and origin. The parathyroid glands are composed of chief cells that secrete parathyroid hormone, which is crucial to calcium homeostasis. The external or cranial parathyroid glands are derived from the third pharyngeal pouch (parathyroid III) while the internal or caudal parathyroids come from the fourth pharyngeal pouch (ultimobranchial body; parathyroid IV).

Necropsy Guide for Dogs, Cats, and Small Mammals, First Edition. Edited by Sean P. McDonough and Teresa Southard.
© 2017 John Wiley & Sons, Inc. Published 2017 by John Wiley & Sons, Inc.
Companion Website: www.wiley.com/go/mcdonough/necropsy

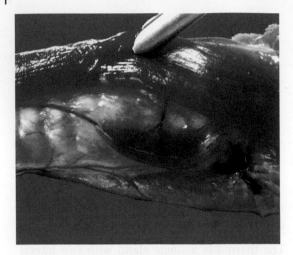

Figure 13.1 Thyroid gland. The thyroid lobes are closely applied to the trachea, just caudal to the larynx.

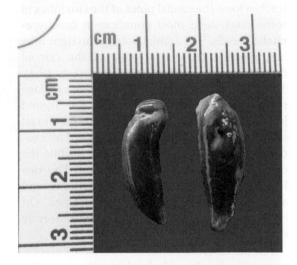

Figure 13.2 Parathyroid glands. The parathyroid glands are intimately associated with the thyroid. The cranial or external parathyroid gland resides at or near the cranial pole of the thyroid lobe. The caudal, or internal, parathyroid gland is typically embedded in the thyroid and can only be found by careful sectioning.

The external parathyroid gland is located on the lateral surface of the cranial half of the thyroid lobe (Fig. 13.2). In 10% of dogs it is on the lateral surface of the caudal half of the lobe. The external parathyroid is usually flat with an ovate outline and the color varies from yellow-brown to yellow-red to golden yellow. In small dogs the gland is 1 mm while in giant breed it can be as large as 7.5 mm. The internal (caudal) parathyroid is typically embedded in the medial surface at the middle of the thyroid lobe. Sometimes the internal parathyroid is located near the caudal pole or along the dorsal edge so careful sectioning of the thyroid may be necessary to locate it. The internal parathyroid glands are generally smaller, rounder, and flatter than the external parathyroids.

13.1.3 The Endocrine Pancreas (Islets of Langerhans)

The endocrine pancreas consists of scattered microscopic islands of endocrine cells known as Islets of Langerhans. The number of islets in the dog is greater in the left limb. The cat pancreas has large Pacinian corpuscles in the interlobular regions and can be visualized as 1–3 mm diameter white foci. These should not be mistaken for Islets of Langerhans.

13.1.4 The Adrenal Glands

The adrenal cortex and medulla are derived from two different origins, although they are considered to represent a single organ. The cortex produces steroid hormones from cholesterol. The outer zona glomerulosa secretes aldosterone primarily in response to angiotensin II (renin-angiotensin-aldosterone axis) but mild, transitory, delayed aldosertone secretion is also stimulated by K^+ and ACTH. The zona fasciculata releases glucocorticoids in response to ACTH. The innermost zona reticularis produces sex hormones (progesterone, estrogens, and androgens) in minute amounts that are most likely of no physiologic importance. The medulla is a sympathetic paraganglion and medullary chromaffin cells synthesize and secrete either epinephrine or norepinephrine.

The adrenal glands are asymmetrical in shape and position. They are flattened, bilobed organs located cranial and medial to the kidneys on either side of the aorta. The right adrenal gland lies opposite the last thoracic or first lumbar

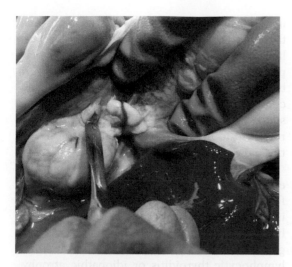

Figure 13.3 Adrenal glands. The adrenal glands are located cranial to the kidneys and are often embedded in fat, making them difficult to visualize. The cranial abdominal (phrenocoabdominal) vein runs in a groove over the ventral surface, aiding in identification. In extremely obese animals, gentle palpation and careful incisions are necessary to locate the adrenals.

vertebra at the level of the cranial mesenteric artery. The left adrenal gland is more caudal than the right, reflecting the more caudal position of the left kidney, and is opposite the second lumbar vertebra. The cranial abdominal (phrenoco-abdominal) vein runs in an oblique groove across the ventral surface of each gland (Fig. 13.3). The right adrenal gland is comma-shaped and is separated from the right crus of the diaphragm by a small amount of adipose tissue. When sectioned, the adrenal cortex is firm and yellowish while the medulla is softer and brown. The normal cortex to medullary ratio is 1:1.

13.2 *In Situ* Evaluation and Removal

13.2.1 The Pituitary Gland

Removal of the brain at necropsy typically ruptures the infundibular stalk, leaving the pituitary gland in the hypophyseal fossa. The dura mater passes over the caudal clinoid processes and around the sides of the pituitary gland

forming an open window in the diaphragma sella. Cysts are common in the adenohypophysis. Most are microscopic, age-associated changes of no significance. If they become very large they may encroach on adjacent structures. The craniopharyngeal duct normally disappears by birth. Cystic remnants of the distal or sellar end of the craniopharyngeal duct are extremely common in brachycephalic breeds of dogs, occurring in about half of dogs with this conformation. The cysts are located at the periphery of the pars distalis and pars tuberalis.

Pituitary gland tumors are most commonly found in dogs and are almost always benign. Microadenomas are as likely to be endocrinologically active as macroadenomas, which necessitates histopathological evaluation for confirmation. Since the diaphragma sellae is incomplete, macroadenomas expand dorsally (supra sellar expansion) causing indentation and compression of the overlying hypothalamus and occasionally the thalamus. Large pituitary gland adenomas are firmly attached to the underlying basisphenoid bone but do not invade or erode the base of the hypophyseal fossa. Growth along the base of the brain may impair the function of the optic, oculomotor and trochlear nerves causing blindness and strabismus.

The only disease of significance of the pars nervosa is primary diabetes insipidus. Destruction of the neurohypophysis can be caused by large pituitary tumors, cysts, abscesses, granulomas, extension of local neoplasms, or metastatic lesions. Trauma seldom causes pituitary dysfunction, probably because head injury of sufficient severity to cause hypothalamic and pituitary damage likely leads to early death.

Metastatic neoplasms to the pituitary gland include lymphoma, melanoma, transmissible venereal tumor and mammary gland adenocarcinomas. Osteosarcoma of the sphenoid bone, ependymoma of the infundibular recess of the third ventricle, gliomas of the infundibular stalk and basilar meningiomas may compress and/or infiltrate the pituitary gland.

Removal of the pituitary gland is greatly facilitated if the dorsum sellae and associated caudal

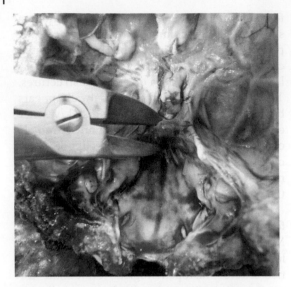

Figure 13.4 Collecting the pituitary gland is difficult since the clinoid process partially covers the caudal aspect. Cutting the clinoid process with a pair of sharp bone forceps greatly facilitates collection and minimizes the chance of damaging the pituitary gland.

clinoid processes are first removed using small, sharp bone forceps (Fig. 13.4). Harvest the pituitary by grasping the fascia around the pituitary gland with rat tooth forceps and use a scalpel blade to dissect the pituitary gland away from the bony hypophyseal fossa.

13.2.2 The Thyroid and Parathyroid Glands

Because the parathyroid glands are intimately associated with the thyroid, these two endocrine organs are assessed concurrently. The thyroid lobes lie in the fascia on either side of the trachea and are as closely attached to the overlying musculature as they are to the trachea. Thus, care must be taken when removing the pluck not to lose the thyroid gland by cutting too closely to the trachea. Compare the left and right lobes for size, color, shape, texture, and consistency. Thyroglossal duct cysts are seen occasionally in the midline cranial cervical region of dogs. Small nodules (1–2 mm) of accessory thyroid tissue can be found anywhere from the base of tongue to the diaphragm (found in 50% of dogs). The nodules retain normal thyroid structure and function but lack parafollicular C-cells. These sites can undergo hyperplasia or become thyroid tumors (e.g., heart base tumor). Thyroid aplasia, hypoplasia, and congenital goiter are rare. Multifocal white spots representing C-cell hyperplasia in response to hypercalcemia may be seen in the thyroid of dogs.

Primary hypothyroidism is the most common endocrinopathy of adult dogs. Any structural or functional derangement that significantly impairs output of hormone (>75%) will cause hypothyroidism. Most affected dogs have progressive loss of thyroid tissue as a result either lymphocytic thyroiditis or idiopathic atrophy. Thyroid carcinomas are common in dogs with up to 75% of dogs greater than 17 years of age affected. Approximately 20% are functional and 15% are bilateral. Half of all dogs with thyroid carcinomas at the time of clinical presentation have metastases. Lymphatic drainage leads to unique patterns of metastasis. Caudal lymphatics bypass lymph nodes and enter the brachiocephalic trunk, resulting in early metastasis to the lungs. Cranial lymphatic drainage is to retropharyngeal lymph nodes. The vast majority of hyperthyroid cats (98%) have adenomatous (multinodular) hyperplasia (Fig. 13.5). Among hyperthyroid cats with thyroid neoplasia, 35% have adenomas and 65% have carcinomas. Affected cats may develop hypertrophic cardiomyopathy due to increased afterload (systemic hypertension) and the trophic effects of thyroid hormone on cardiomyocytes.

Remnants of the third and fourth pharyngeal pouches often form small, multiloculated cysts in or near the parathyroids of dogs. Their location helps distinguish them from thyroglossal duct cysts, which are located on the midline. Agenesis of the parathyroid glands is recognized as a rare cause of hypoparathyroidism in puppies.

Parathyroid or chief cell adenomas are seen infrequently in older dogs and cats and are not a consequence of long standing secondary hyperparathyroidism (Fig. 13.6). A single gland is typically affected but bilateral parathyroid

Figure 13.5 Feline hyperthoroidism. The vast majority of hyperthyroid cats have multinodular (adenomatous) hyperplasia.

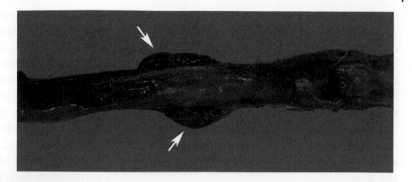

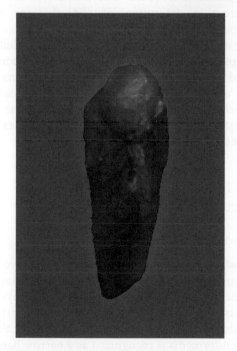

Figure 13.6 Parathyroid gland (chief cell) adenoma. An adenoma is a solitary, sharply demarcated, expansile mass. Parathyroid gland hyperplasia affects all parathyroid glands bilaterally.

adenomas have been reported rarely. Parathyroid carcinomas are less frequent, generally larger than adenomas and are fixed in position due to invasion of adjacent tissues. If the parathyroid tumor is functional, it results in primary hyperparathyroidism. Long standing cases of primary hyperparathyroidism may have osteopenia with pathologic fractures, facial hyperostosis leading to partial obstruction of

the nasal cavity and loosening or loss of teeth. Parathyroid tissue adjacent to an adenoma undergoes pressure atrophy. If the tumor is functional, the remaining chief cells are atrophied due to negative feedback inhibition from persistent hypercalcemia. These changes are difficult or impossible to appreciate grossly.

Parathyroid gland hyperplasia affects multiple glands, which helps to distinguish this from an adenoma. Idiopathic primary hyperparathyroidism, with enlargement of all parathyroid glands, is most often encountered in Keeshonds, suggesting a genetic cause. Secondary hyperparathyroidism also leads to hyperplasia of all parathyroid glands and when encountered, a detailed dietary history and thorough evaluation of the kidneys is indicated. Fibrous osteodystrophy may be encountered in long standing cases.

13.2.3 The Endocrine Pancreas

Since the islets of Langerhans are microscopic, evaluation is generally accomplished by histopathology. Diabetes mellitus is most common in dogs and encountered less frequently in cats. Affected dogs are typically older with females affected more often than males. In cats, diabetes also affects older cats most often but the incidence is higher in males than females. Necrotizing pancreatitis is the most common cause of diabetes mellitus in dogs with islet tissue destroyed secondary to inflammatory disease of the exocrine pancreas. Most diabetic cats have insulin resistance with obesity as the major risk factor. Prolonged overstimulation of the beta cells in diabetic cats often leads to deposition of amyloid in the islets but is unlikely to be recognized grossly.

Islet cell tumors are encountered on occasion and may be functional (e.g., "insulinoma"). Islet cell tumors are pale, grey-purple, firm, sharply demarcated masses located anywhere in the pancreas. Their typically bland gross appearance belies the fact that most are carcinomas and metastasize to regional lymph nodes and the liver.

13.2.4 The Adrenal Glands

The hepatorenal ligament is variable in occurrence but when present extends from the medial aspect of the renal fossa in the caudate process to the ventral surface of the right kidney. The right adrenal gland is situated just dorsal to the ligament. The cranial abdominal (phrenicoabdominal) vein runs in a groove across the ventral surface of the adrenal glands and is reliable landmark. In postmortem cases, the left adrenal gland it often lies beneath the caudal vena cava. The caudal lobes of both the left and right adrenals are embedded in fat but in obese animals, the entire adrenal gland is completely hidden from view. In this case, carefully palpate and incise the fat cranial to the kidneys until the glands are located.

Unilateral agenesis, most commonly on the left side, occurs occasionally. Cortical adenomas are typically uniformly light yellow and tend to be encapsulated as compared to cortical nodular hyperplasia. Carcinomas are larger, more likely to be bilateral and may be variegated yellow-red due to hemorrhage and necrosis. If the masses are functional, contralateral adrenocortical atrophy is expected. Other hyperfunctional syndromes are rare but include hyperandrogenism (adrenogenital syndrome, adrenal virilism), hyperestrogenism, and hyperprogesteronism. Hyperaldosteronism due to a tumor of the zona glomerulosa (Conn's syndrome) is seen rarely in cats. Glucocorticoid administration causes bilateral cortical atrophy whereas a functional chromophobe adenoma (excess ACTH) leads to bilateral cortical hyperplasia.

Primary hypoadrenocorticism (Addison's-like Disease) is occasionally encountered in dogs but is rare in cats. Idiopathic immune-mediated destruction of all zones of the cortex is most common. Treatment with op'DDD destroys the zona fasciculata and zona reticularis but usually spares the zona glomerulosa. In long standing cases, macronodular regeneration may lead to drug resistance and recurrence of clinical signs. Because of the rich blood supply, metastatic carcinomas, and spread of infection to the adrenal glands is frequent. The amount of tissue destruction determines if clinical signs of hypoadrenocorticism develop.

Several neoplasms arise in the adrenal medulla but pheochromocytoma is the only one encountered with any regularity. Pheochromocytomas are usually non-functional but may release catecholamines sporadically. These tumors have a high propensity to invade the posterior vena cava but rarely generate distant metastases.

13.3 Organ Examination, Sectioning, and Fixation

13.3.1 The Pituitary Gland

Grossly, the pars nervosa is a spherical to ovoid extension of the infundibulum. The pars distalis is the largest portion of the adenohypophysis and is separated from the pars intermedia by the residual Rathke's cleft. On close inspection, the pars intermedia is recognized as a narrow band of dark tissue on the dorsal wall of Rathke's cleft and intimately associated with the surface of the pars nervosa. The pars tuberalis is also dark, owing to the rich hypophyseal portal blood supply, and appears as an extension of the pars distalis closely applied to the surface of the infundibular stalk. Visualization of these relationships is greatly aided by the use of a dissecting microscope or magnifying lens.

The pituitary gland is best sectioned after fixation and it is most convenient to forward the intact gland in formalin to the pathologist. Incise the gland along the midline and examine the cut surface. Cut one side transversely and

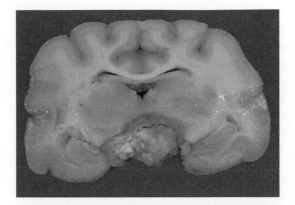

Figure 13.7 Pituitary gland carcinoma. The pituitary gland has been obliterated and the neoplastic pituicytes have infiltrated adjacent structures.

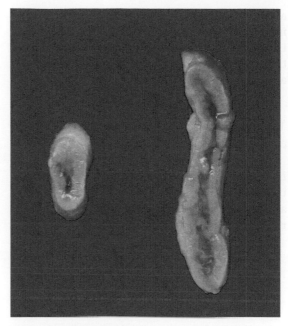

Figure 13.8 Adrenal glands. The normal cortex to medulla ratio is 1:1. A transverse section of the right adrenal and a longitudinal section of the left aids in identification when trimming.

submit all three sections for histopathological evaluation. If suspecting a microadenoma (e.g., corticotroph adenoma) be sure to indicate this since the block will need to be step-sectioned in order to find a small mass. Rare pituitary carcinomas obliterate the gland and invade adjacent structures (Fig. 13.7).

13.3.2 The Thyroid and Parathyroid Glands

Normally the thyroids and parathyroids are small enough to be placed whole in fixative. A transverse cut through the right lobe into cranial and caudal halves facilitates identification. Alternatively, they can be submitted in cassettes labelled with a number 2 lead pencil.

13.3.3 The Endocrine Pancreas

Make parallel transverse slices ("bread-loafing") every 1–2 cm through both the left and right lobes and collect representative samples. Samples from both the left and right lobes as well as any lesions should be taken. Leaving a section of duodenum attached to the right lobe aids in identification.

13.3.4 The Adrenal Glands

After harvesting the adrenal glands, evaluate the cortical to medullary ratio. The normal ratio is 1:1 but can be easily skewed if the slice is even slightly oblique. Cut the right adrenal gland transversely and the left longitudinally to aid in identification (Fig. 13.8).

Accessory adrenal cortical tissue is frequent in the adrenal capsule of dogs but less frequent in cats. Nodular hyperplasia is a common, incidental necropsy finding, especially in old dogs. Hyperplastic nodules may involve any of the three zones of the cortex, are usually multiple, bilateral, and appear as sharply demarcated but unencapsulated and non-expansile nodules in the cortex or attached to the capsule. Nodular hyperplasia of the zona reticularis imparts an irregular contour to the corticomedullary junction. Mineralized necrotic cortical tissue that extends into the medulla is present in about one third of cats but in only about 5% of dogs. The change can be extensive but regenerative nodular hyperplasia prevents clinical signs.

Pheochromocytomas are variegated light brown to yellow-red due to areas of necrosis and hemorrhage. The Henle chromoreaction can be a valuable aid in distinguishing cortical carcinomas from pheochromocytomas. Zenker's solution, which oxidizes catecholamines, applied to the cut surface of a freshly resected tumor forms a dark brown pigment within 20 min.

13.4 Common Artifacts and Postmortem Changes

Due to the rich blood supply and high metabolic rate, endocrine organs autolyze rapidly. Collection and immersion in fixative as quickly as possible is recommended.

Rough handling when collecting adrenals can cause extrusion of the medulla creating a pseudocystic change with a central cavity that can be blood filled. Streaks of cortical hemorrhage are common in newborns (birth trauma). Increased peripheral resistance as an animal dies can cause agonal hemorrhages in the adrenal gland so care must be taken not to over interpret adrenal hemorrhages.

Release of lysosomal enzymes due to autolysis can lead to breakdown of blood vessels and postmortem leakage of blood into the pancreas (see Fig. 9.7). This must not be confused with necrohemorrhagic pancreatitis.

14

The Lymphoreticular System

14.1 Anatomy Review

14.1.1 Thymus

The primary function of the thymus is to produce T-lymphocytes. The thymus is derived from the third pharyngeal pouches as epithelial outgrowths that merge on the midline. In dogs and cats, the thymic anlage then migrates caudally to the mediastinum just cranial to the heart. In puppies and kittens, the thymus is roughly triangular, laterally compressed, and located in the precardial mediastinal septum. In fresh carcasses, the thymus has a pink tinge that rapidly fades to grey with autolysis (Fig. 14.1). Distinct right and left lobes are visible caudally but are merged cranially. The thymus has a lobulated structure and each lobule may measure over 1 cm. The lobules are separated by delicate fibrous trabeculae that allow them to move freely on each other.

14.1.2 Lymph Nodes

The lymph nodes filter antigen and infectious agents from the afferent lymph and produce efferent lymph rich in antibody and lymphocytes. Lymph nodes are situated where they are protected by the surrounding tissue but produce minimum interference with the function of the musculoskeletal and vascular systems. Thus, they are usually located in fat stores at the flexor angles of joints, in the mediastinum and mesentery, and at the angle formed by the origin of many of the larger blood vessels.

Each lymph node drains a reasonably well defined area of regional anatomy but extensive anastomosis is present so drainage areas overlap. Lymphocenters consist of a single lymph node or a group of lymph nodes that occur constantly in the same region of the body and receive afferent lymphatics from approximately the same regions in all species: (1) Head (mandibular, parotid, and retropharyngeal lymph nodes), (2) Cervical (superficial and deep cervical lymph nodes), (3) Thoracic limb (axillary lymph node), (4) Thoracic cavity (dorsal and ventral thoracic lymph nodes, mediastinal lymph nodes, and tracheobronchial lymph nodes), (5) Abdominal and pelvic wall (lumbar, iliosacral, inguinofemoral, and ischiatic lymph nodes), (6) Abdominal viscera (celiac, cranial mesenteric, caudal mesenteric lymph nodes), and (7) Distal pelvic limb (popliteal lymph node).

The afferent lymphatics enter the subcapsular sinus and drain into the medullary sinuses that converge at the hilus to form efferent lymphatics. Efferent lymphatics eventually return tissue fluid and leukocytes to the venous blood supply via the thoracic duct that enters the great vessels of the heart, usually near the junction of the left external jugular vein and the cranial vena cava. On section, a lymph node has a fibrous capsule and a poorly defined cortex and medulla (Fig. 14.2).

14.1.3 Spleen

The spleen is an elongated organ that is roughly triangular in cross-section. It lies in the left

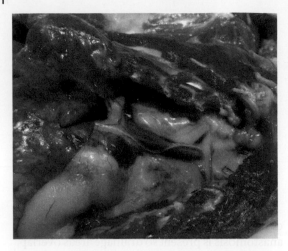

Figure 14.1 Thymus in a young adult cat. The thymus begins to involute around 4–5 months of age in most dogs and cats. If the thymic remnant is not visible, an *en bloc* resection of the cranial mediastinum to include the cranial pericardial sac will reliably include the thymus.

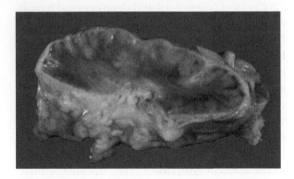

Figure 14.2 Lymph node. Lymph nodes are usually embedded in abundant adipose tissue. On cut surface the capsule is a thin band of fibrous connective tissue. The cortex and medulla are ill defined but the cortex is usually grey-white, bulges on section, and may be nodular (follicular hyperplasia). The medulla is usually darker than the cortex.

hypogastric region and roughly parallels the greater curvature of the stomach. The spleen is loosely attached to the greater curvature of the stomach by the gastrosplenic ligament, which is part of the greater omentum. The dorsal end or head of the spleen is rounded, wedge-shaped and lies between the gastric fundus and the cranial pole of the left kidney (Fig. 14.3). The ventral end or tail is more variable in both shape

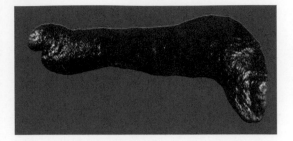

Figure 14.3 Spleen. The dorsal end (head of the spleen is rounded and wedge-shaped while the ventral end (tail) is generally wider. When contracted, the capsular surface is grey-brown with a purple cast but when congested is dark red-purple.

and location, but is generally wider. When contracted, the capsular surface is grey-brown with a purple cast but when congested is dark red-purple. The splenic artery arises as a branch of the celiac artery and divides into a dorsal and ventral branch. These branches give rise to up to approximately 25 splenic branches that penetrate the capsule at the longitudinal hilus along the visceral surface. The venous outflow parallels the arterial inflow and empties into the portal vein.

Splenic architecture is complex with precise localization of leukocyte subsets to different micro environments resulting in functional compartmentalization. As splenic arterioles leave the smooth muscle trabeculae, they become surrounded by T-cells that form periarteriolar lymphoid sheaths. B-cells form primary and secondary follicles near the nodular arterioles, analogous to follicles in lymph nodes. Completely surrounding these T- and B-cell domains is the marginal zone, which forms the interface between the red pulp and the white pulp. No post capillary high endothelial venules or afferent lymphatics are present in the spleen and lymphocyte trafficking occurs through the marginal zone. In addition, marginal zone macrophages participate in the inductive phases of antibody responses by efficiently processing and presenting particulate antigens to T-cells and B-cells that traffic through the region. The red pulp consists of sinuses sandwiched between red pulp cords. While the spleen has efferent lymphatics, no afferent lymphatics are present and antigen gains access to either the red pulp or the white pulp via the marginal zones. Thus, the spleen is an "in-line" filter of blood but is relatively protected from exposure to antigen when compared to lymph nodes.

Macrophages in the red pulp cords function in defense against bacterial sepsis by opsonized phagocytosis mediated by both Fc and complement fragment receptors. Additional red pulp functions include maturation of reticulocytes, pitting of erythrocytes, and removal of senescent cells. The red pulp is not merely a filtration bed with phagocytic macrophages but also contains unique populations of lymphocytes. Finally, the red pulp stores significant numbers of erythrocytes and platelets. Splenic contraction can deliver a significant "autoinfusion" to help counter the effects of acute hemorrhage or during intense bouts of exercise.

14.1.4 Bone Marrow

Depending on the amount of hematopoietic and adipose tissue, bone marrow is classified as either red marrow or yellow marrow. Red marrow predominates in the flat bones of the skull, ribs, sternum, and pelvis as well as in the epiphysis and metaphysis of long bones. Yellow marrow is found in the diaphysis of long bones. The cellularity of bone marrow varies by age. In adolescents, 75% of the marrow consists of hematopoietic cells with the number declining to 50% in adults, and 25% in geriatric animals. In adults, most red marrow is present in the flat bones, vertebral bodies, and metaphyses of long bones.

14.2   *In Situ* Evaluation and Removal

14.2.1   Thymus

The thymus grows rapidly during the first few months of life and reaches maximum size between 4 and 5 months of age. Thymic involution begins around the time the deciduous incisors are shed. As the thymus involutes, it is replaced by fat. Involution is accelerated by

severe stress and the degree of thymic involution is a rough index of the severity and duration of disease in young animals. Importantly, although the thymus never completely disappears, the thymic remnant is rarely visible in adults. Resection of the cranial pericardial sac and the cranial mediastinal septum ventral to the trachea will reliably include the thymic remnant.

Thymic hypoplasia can be seen in congenital immunodeficiency syndromes (e.g., severe combined immunodeficiency) while thymic atrophy can be seen with acquired immunodeficiency states. Thymic cysts are relatively common but are generally small and incidental lesions in older dogs.

Thymic enlargement may rarely reflect diffuse hyperplasia but most often is due either to thymic lymphoma or thymoma. Both are space occupying masses that displace the lungs dorsally and may infiltrate around the great vessels of the heart. Thymomas are irregularly shaped with a firm, fibrous capsule that gives rise to thick fibrous septations that subdivide the parenchyma (Fig. 14.4). In contrast, thymic

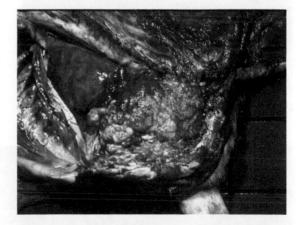

Figure 14.4 Thymoma. Lymphomas and thymomas account for the vast majority of cranial mediastinal neoplasms. Both are space occupying and displace the lungs dorsally. The masses may infiltrate around the great vessels of the heart. Thymomas are characterized by a firm, fibrous capsule that gives rise to thick fibrous septations that subdivide the parenchyma. In contrast, thymic lymphomas are poorly encapsulated, traversed by fine, irregular fibrous septa with a homogenous cut surface that bulges.

lymphomas are poorly encapsulated and traversed by fine, irregular fibrous septa. Rarely, other tumors such as primary germ cell neoplasms and neuroendocrine carcinomas arise in the mediastinum.

14.2.2 Lymph Nodes

Lymphoid depletion accompanies a wide variety of systemic disease states but this can seldom be appreciated grossly. Thus, gross evaluation of lymph nodes is primarily restricted to detecting lymphadenomegaly (Fig. 14.5). Care should be taken not to over interpret the size of lymph nodes in young animals as they are typically enlarged compared to their adult counterparts. Since lymph nodes are usually embedded in fat,

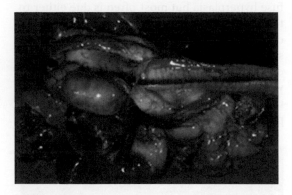

Figure 14.5 Multicentric lymphoma. Generalized lymphadenomegaly with non-painful lymph nodes fixed to the surrounding tissue is the most common presentation of lymphoma.

gentle palpation and careful incisions will help locate and isolate lymph nodes. Lymph node enlargement may be due to reactive hyperplasia, inflammation, or neoplasia. Since each lymph node drains a reasonably well defined area of regional anatomy, the drainage field should be inspected for evidence of infection, hemorrhage, necrosis, trauma, or neoplasia.

14.2.3 Spleen

The spleen is most easily harvested by preserving its attachments to the stomach and removing it with the rest of the alimentary system. After the alimentary tract is exteriorized, incise the gastrosplenic ligament to free the spleen from the stomach. Evaluate the size, shape, color, and consistency paying particular attention to any masses. The spleen is ruptured fairly easily in dogs and cats hit by cars (Fig. 14.6). The spleen may be fully divided into two or more parts or it may simply rupture and heal by scarring. Traumatic rupture of the spleen can result in implants of splenic parenchyma in the omentum where they survive and form "accessory" spleens.

Animals euthanized with barbiturates generally have an enlarged, congested spleen. Otherwise, an enlarged spleen is almost invariably a diseased spleen.

14.2.3.1 Red Pulp

Diffuse enlargement of the spleen is generally due to changes in the red pulp. Spleens enlarged for any reason are prone to thrombosis and

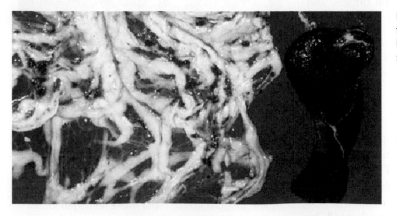

Figure 14.6 Fractured spleen. The fracture lines have healed with linear scars. Note the implants of splenic tissue on the omentum.

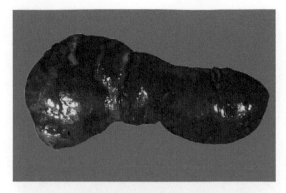

Figure 14.7 Splenic infarcts. Splenomegaly of any cause predisposes the spleen to infarction due to sluggish blood flow that fails to sweep activated clotting factors out of the spleen.

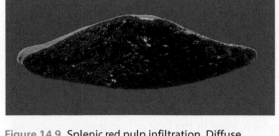

Figure 14.9 Splenic red pulp infiltration. Diffuse expansion of the splenic red pulp by extramedullary hematopoiesis, red pulp macrophage hyperplasia or infiltration by hematopoietic neoplasia creates a spleen with a "meaty" consistency that is dry and dark red on section.

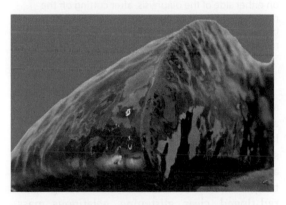

Figure 14.8 Splenic congestion. A congested spleen has a pulpy consistency and oozes thick, red-black blood from the cut surface.

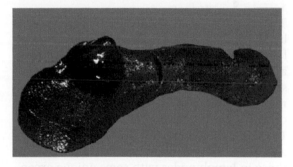

Figure 14.10 Splenic hemangiosarcoma. The bulk of a splenic hemangiosarcoma is a hematoma with only a thin band of neoplastic tissue around the margin. Multiple sections (6–8) form around the periphery of the mass will reliably distinguish a benign hematoma from hemangiosarcoma.

infarction (Fig. 14.7). Diffusely enlarged spleens can be further subdivided into those that are "pulpy" versus those that are "meaty". Pulpy spleens are congested and when sectioned, the surface oozes thick, red-black blood (Fig. 14.8). Thrombosis of the splenic vein, splenic torsion and gastric dilatation volvulus are the most common causes of splenic congestion.

A fleshy to firm consistency in an enlarged spleen indicates diffuse red pulp involvement. On section the spleen has a dry, dark red surface (Fig. 14.9). Red pulp macrophage hyperplasia arises in response to prolonged particulate anti-genemia such as blood borne parasites or chronic hemolytic anemia. Myeloid metaplasia

occurs when the bone marrow is unable to meet demands for increased cell production but the proper stimuli for hematopoiesis and pluripotent hematopoietic stem cells remain in the circulation. Induction of extramedullary hematopoiesis occurs under a wide variety of circumstances including bone marrow failure and chronic anemia (especially hemolytic anemia). Myelopoiesis predominates in infectious toxemias, such as pyometra in the bitch. Lastly, leukemias of all types may infiltrate the splenic sinusoids as a secondary site of involvement.

A variety of sarcomas arise in the splenic red pulp. Hemangiosarcoma (Fig. 14.10) is most frequent but must be differentiated from splenic hematomas, which usually arise in foci of nodular hyperplasia. Leiomyosarcomas and myxosarcomas, along with their benign counterparts, are encountered occasionally. Disseminated histiocytic sarcoma (malignant histiocytosis) can often involve the spleen.

Metastatic carcinomas are seldom found in the spleen, even in the face of hematogenous spread. The reason for this is uncertain but may reflect efficient killing of neoplastic cells by resident macrophages and lymphocytes. Alternatively, the spleen may not provide an environment that can sustain growth of neoplastic epithelial cells.

14.2.3.2 White Pulp

The spleen is relatively sheltered from antigen by the innate immune system, while regional lymph nodes and Kupffer cells efficiently filter antigen. Thus, reactive hyperplasia in the splenic white pulp implies systemic antigenemia. Lymphoid hyperplasia manifests as numerous, randomly distributed, soft, white nodules 1–2 mm in diameter. Hematopoietic neoplasms arising in the spleen are generally analogous to those in lymph nodes with some unique exceptions (e.g., hepatosplenic lymphoma and large granular lymphocytic leukemia).

14.2.4 Bone Marrow

At necropsy, bone marrow can be collected from the costochondral junction, the sternum, or a vertebral body. However, bone marrow is most easily collected from the metaphysis of a long bone. The femur can be cracked, as described in Chapter 3 to harvest bone marrow. Alternatively, all the marrow from the diaphysis can be collected with a with a longitudinal section. First, cut off the proximal and distal metaphyses of a long bone with a bone saw. Next, make two deep longitudinal score lines on either side of the diaphysis with an oscillating saw. Use a stout pair of bone forceps to crack the diaphysis in half and harvest the core of yellow fat, being sure to include red marrow at the metaphysis (Fig. 14.11).

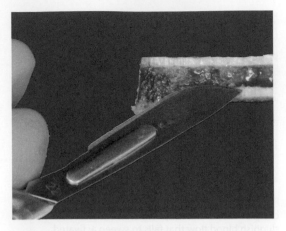

Figure 14.11 Bone marrow. Rather than cracking a bone with rib cutters, two deep score lines can be made on either side of the diaphysis, after cutting off the metaphyses, and then cracking the bone with a pair of bone forceps. Use a scalpel blade to harvest bone marrow.

Gross evaluation of bone marrow is limited to assessing the amount and distribution of red and yellow marrow. In leukemias, neoplastic hematopoietic cells can extend over the outer surface of the diaphyseal core of yellow marrow as a thin, light brown layer. In emaciated animals, the yellow marrow is transformed into a grey- or red-tinged, clear, glistening, gelatinous mass, termed serous atrophy of fat (Fig. 14.12).

14.3 Organ Examination, Sectioning, and Fixation

14.3.1 Thymus

Collect a representative of any lesions and fix by immersion in 10% neutral buffered formalin.

14.3.2 Lymph Nodes

Dissect as much fat away from the lymph node as possible before sectioning. Impression smears may identify bacteria, fungi, protozoa, or neoplastic cells (see Chapter 17). Small lymph nodes (up to 3 mm thick) are best submitted whole. Larger lymph nodes are bisected on the

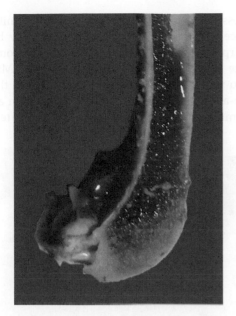

Figure 14.12 Serous atrophy of fat. Evaluation of yellow fat in the diaphysis is an important part of assessing an emaciated animal. Serous atrophy of fat converts the adipose to a clear, grey to red-tinged, gelatinous, glistening mass.

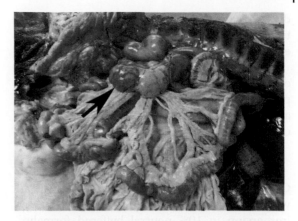

Figure 14.13 Canine lymphoma. Note the enlarged mesenteric lymph node at the root of the mesentery (arrow).

long axis to include both cortex and medulla. If necessary, further slices every 2–3 mm are made. Inspect the surface for obvious abnormalities (e.g., loss of distinction between cortex and medulla, tumor infiltration, etc.). Since lymph nodes filter and concentrate antigen, they are an excellent specimen for bacteriology and virology. Collect samples in appropriate transport media.

Lymphadenitis occurs when an infectious agent or inflammatory products (fluids and cells) drain into the node from a distant site. The type of inflammatory response can provide important clues to the nature of the disease even if a specific agent is not seen. Acute lymphadenitis will have neutrophilic infiltrates. Necrosis and liquefaction with abscess formation or caseation are possible depending on host/agent factors. In contrast, rapid lysis and lymphocyte depletion with very little inflammatory response is characteristic of some acute viral infections (feline and canine parvovirus infection).

Lymph nodes with chronic lymphadenitis are enlarged and firm. These nodes are often dominated by reactive hyperplastic changes, and medullary cords may be expanded by plasma cells. The connective tissue septa and capsule may be thickened by fibrosis. Extracellular (higher bacteria and fungi) or intracellular infectious agents (e.g., Leishmania, *Histoplasma capsulatum*, *Neorickettsia salmincola*) may be recognizable.

The most common neoplasm in lymph nodes is lymphosaracoma (Fig. 14.13). Lymphomatous lymph nodes are enlarged and "fixed" to the surrounding tissue because of invasion of the capsule by neoplastic lymphocytes. The node is soft or fleshy in consistency, grey-white, and bulges from the cut surface. Leukemias often extend to lymph nodes as secondary sites of involvement. In advanced disease, total lymph node effacement and perinodal infiltration occurs and distinguishing a case of lymphoma from leukemia is difficult. Examination of bone marrow and peripheral blood are usually more diagnostic in these cases.

Because lymph nodes filter the cells and fluids that gain access to interstitial tissues, metastatic neoplasms often spread via lymphatic vessels to regional lymph nodes. Metastases usually colonize the subcapsular sinus and then expand to eventually involve the entire node. Extension downstream to the next lymph node and eventually to the lungs via peripheral blood is the expected pattern of tumor metastasis.

Fixation by immersion in 10% neutral buffered formalin is sufficient. B5 provides excellent preservation of nuclear detail, but the expense and toxicity are not justified in the vast majority of cases.

14.3.3 Spleen

Collect representative samples of any lesions as well as normal appearing spleen and fix by immersion in 10% neutral buffered formalin. Large splenic masses, such as hemangiosarcoma (Fig. 14.10), can be problematic since the volume of fixative needed is impractical and penetration will not occur before the center of the lesion is autolyzed. Inspection slices can help with penetration but unless done carefully, can make it difficult for the pathologist to identify margins. In this situation, consider placing the intact spleen in a leak-proof plastic bag, wrapping the bag in several layers of newspaper or paper towel to prevent freezing and ship it overnight with a sufficient number of frozen gel packs to keep the contents cool. The pathologist can then select appropriate samples. Alternatively, collect 6–8 sections from around the circumference of the mass spanning the margin with adjacent normal parenchyma and place in an appropriate volume of formalin. Submission of an annotated digital image with the sections labelled according to location is a great aid to the pathologist when evaluating the sections histologically.

14.3.4 Bone Marrow

Complete evaluation of bone marrow requires both histopathology and cytology (see Fig. 17.2). Histopathology of decalcified metaphyseal bone allows for evaluation of trabecular bone, blood vessels, bone marrow stroma, and can provide an indication of cellularity. However, morphologic changes, altered myeloid to erythroid (M:E) ratio, and abnormalities in proliferation or maturation of hematopoietic cells are best

assessed cytologically. Importantly, the significance of the cytological findings can only be interpreted in light of a contemporaneous complete blood count. For example, a normal M:E ratio with normal cellularity is expected in the non-anemic state but is hyporegenerative in an anemic animal with no peripheral reticulocytes.

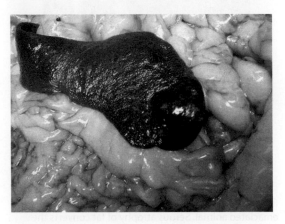

Figure 14.14 Partial splenic congestion. Animal euthanized in extremis may have only partial areas of splenic congestion that must not be confused with splenic infarcts.

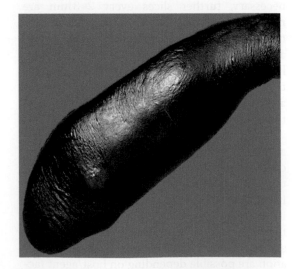

Figure 14.15 Splenic nodular hyperplasia. Nodules of hyperplastic white pulp are common in the spleen of older dogs. Histopathology is needed to distinguish these benign mass form a variety of sarcomas that can arise in the spleen.

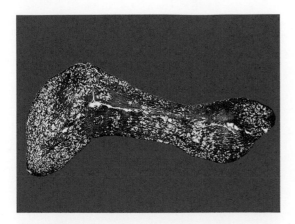

Figure 14.16 Siderotic plaques on the capsule of a dog spleen. These golden brown crusty patches are common incidental lesions in the dog spleen and represent areas of capsular fibrosis mixed with blood breakdown pigments and mineralization.

14.4 Incidental Findings

A variety of changes can be seen in spleens that are of no pathological significance. Animals euthanized in extremis may have only partial areas of splenic congestion (Fig 14.14) that need to be differentiated from splenic infarcts (Fig. 14.7). On occasion, the tail of the spleen is bilobed, which needs to be differentiated from a healed splenic fracture. Nodular hyperplasia (Fig. 14.15) is common in dogs and must be differentiated from a variety of tumors that arise in the spleen. Siderotic plaques are seen commonly in the capsule of canine spleen as golden brown crusty patches that are areas of capsular fibrosis mixed with blood breakdown pigments and mineralization (Fig. 14.16).

Part III

Special Cases

15

Small Mammal Necropsies

Much of the information in this book can also be applied to species other than cats and dogs, such as rabbits, ferrets, guinea pigs, chinchillas, rats, hamsters, gerbils, and mice. This chapter will offer suggestions for modifying the necropsy technique and organ sampling strategy to facilitate postmortem examination of these pocket pets, and review some anatomic peculiarities of each species.

15.1 Species Differences

Most pocket pets, including mice, rats, gerbils, hamsters, guinea pigs, and chinchillas, are members of the order Rodentia. Rabbits are in a separate order, Lagomorpha, but share many features with the rodents. Ferrets are carnivores (order Carnivora), more closely related to dogs and cats than to the other small mammals discussed here. Tables 15.1 and 15.2 highlight some of the characteristic features of these species that may be useful when performing a necropsy.

15.2 Necropsy Technique

The smaller the animal being necropsied, the more we rely on histopathology to identify lesions; however, gross examination is still a very important part of the diagnostic process. Optimal evaluation of even the smallest rodent involves a complete gross examination. The upside of a small animal necropsy is that almost all the tissue can be saved in formalin without violating the 10:1 formalin to tissue ratio.

The external examination in rodents and rabbits should always include a thorough examination of the teeth (Fig. 15.1). Because these species have continuously erupting, or elodont, teeth (incisors in rabbits, rats, mice, gerbils, and hamsters; incisors and cheek teeth in guinea pigs and chinchillas), malocclusion or a low fiber diet can lead to overgrowth of the teeth, inability to properly masticate, damage to surrounding soft tissue, and decreased food intake. Overgrowth of the cheek teeth in guinea pigs and chinchillas results in elongation of the roots and bony nodules along the mandible and maxilla.

In a large rabbit, the necropsy technique described for dogs and cats is appropriate. In smaller animals, the body weight is not sufficient to stabilize the body while the organs are being removed, and the best solution to this problem is to place the body in dorsal recumbency on a cork or Styrofoam cutting board and pin the feet down using insect pins, hypodermic needles, or even thumb tacks (Fig. 15.2). This approach is also useful for young kittens and puppies. The necropsy technique is then modified slightly for this dorsal approach. The skin is opened along the ventral midline and reflected laterally (Fig. 15.3). Alternatively, in mice, gerbils and hamsters, the skin can be completely removed by incising the skin at the umbilicus and around the "waist" and then degloving the skin cranially and caudally, cutting around the

Necropsy Guide for Dogs, Cats, and Small Mammals, First Edition. Edited by Sean P. McDonough and Teresa Southard.
© 2017 John Wiley & Sons, Inc. Published 2017 by John Wiley & Sons, Inc.
Companion Website: www.wiley.com/go/mcdonough/necropsy

Table 15.1 Lifespan, gestation length, litter size and age of sexual maturity in mice, rats, hamsters, gerbils, guinea pigs, chinchillas, and ferrets.

	Lifespan	Gestation	Litter Size	Sexual Maturity
Mouse	2 years	19–21 days	10–12 pups	6 weeks (F) 7–8 weeks (M)
Rat	3–4 years	21–23 days	6–12 pups	4–5 weeks
Hamster	2–3 years	16–22 days	6–8 pups	4–6 weeks
Gerbil	3–4 years	19 days	3–9 pups	9–12 weeks
Guinea Pig	4–5 years	59–73 days	2–4 pups	8–10 weeks (F) 12–14 weeks (M)
Chinchilla	8–10 years	111 days	2–3 kits	7–10 months
Rabbit	9 years	31–33 days	4–12 kits	3.5–4 months (small breeds) 4–4.5 months (medium to large breeds) 6–9 months (giant breeds)
Ferret	5–6 years	42 days	6–10 kits	8–12 months

anus, eyes, and ears (Fig. 15.4). Both coxofemoral joints are easily accessible for opening and examination, and skin, muscle and nerve can be collected as described for the cat and dog. The abdominal body wall is cut along the ventral midline and following the costal margins and reflected laterally (Fig. 15.5). The diaphragm is punctured and then separated from the ribs, which are cut along the ventrolateral aspects (Fig. 15.6). Ribs can be cut with sturdy scissors in mice, gerbils, and hamsters, or with small bone forceps in larger animals. Unlike dogs and cats, rabbits and rodents have bony clavicles that will also need to be cut as the thoracic cavity is opened.

Using a needle and syringe, formalin can be injected into the trachea, to insufflate the lungs (Fig. 15.7), and into the gastrointestinal tract (0.1–0.2 ml at 4–5 sites to avoid damaging the epithelium; Fig. 15.8). This injection technique expands the airways and alveolar spaces and aids in the fixation of the gastrointestinal tract. However, samples should be collected for ancillary tests, if desired, before injection of formalin.

Removal of the pluck, gastrointestinal tract, liver, spleen, and urogenital tract can proceed as in cats and dogs or all of the viscera can be removed as a single unit ("superpluck" or "megapluck"). Start by splitting the mandibular symphysis using scissors and grasp the tongue with forceps (Fig. 15.9). Cut the soft tissue lateral to the tongue, the fascia dorsal to the trachea and esophagus, and the neurovascular bundles going to the forelimbs. Cut the fascia dorsal to the lungs and the diaphragm at the periphery and then undermine the abdominal viscera (Fig. 15.10). The pelvis can be split by inserting closed scissor into the pelvis and opening them (Fig. 15.11). Cut around the anus to free the organs (Fig. 15.12).

Separate and examine the organs. Scissors or small bone forceps are used to open the cranial vault, along approximately the same trajectory as described in cats and dogs, and the brain can be removed and fixed. Alternatively, in mice, hamsters, and gerbils, the entire head can be skinned, fixed, and decalcified for sectioning. Make sure the skin is completely removed or the fixative will not efficiently penetrate the tissue. This whole head technique allows for *in situ* examination of eyes, brain, lacrimal glands, teeth, nasal mucosa, middle and inner ears, and pituitary gland. Transverse cuts on either side of

Table 15.2 Anatomic features of small mammals.

	Mice, Rats, Hamsters, Gerbils	Guinea Pigs, Chinchillas	Rabbits	Ferrets
Teeth	Incisors grow continuously	Incisors and cheek teeth grow continuously	Incisors grow continuously, born with deciduous teeth	Carnivore dentition, teeth do not continuously erupt
Dental Formula	I1/1 C0/0 P0/0 M3/3	I1/1 C0/0 P1/1 M3/3	I2/1 c0/0 P3/2 M3/3	I3/3 C1/1 P3/3 M1/2
Gastrointestinal Tract	Large cecum, squamous and glandular parts of the stomach	Large cecum, simple stomach	Large cecum, simple stomach aboral end of ileum is thickened to form the sacculus rotundus	Short, simple stomach, no cecum, division between jejunum, ileum and colon is indistinct
Liver	Large left lateral lobe, a medial lobe, and small caudate and right lobes Rats do not have a gall bladder	Right lateral, right medial, left lateral, left medial, caudate, quadrate	Left lobe, subdivided into lateral and medial parts, a right lobe, a caudate lobe with caudate and papillary processes and a quadrate lobe	Left lateral, left medial, quadrate, right medial, right lateral and caudate lobes
Lungs	Four right lung lobes (cranial, middle, caudal and accessory) and one left lung lobe	Four right lung lobes (cranial, middle, caudal and accessory) and three left lung lobes (cranial, middle, and caudal)	Four right lung lobes (cranial, middle, caudal and accessory) and two left lung lobes (cranial, middle, and caudal)	Four right lung lobes (cranial, middle, caudal and accessory) Two left lung lobes (cranial and caudal)
Mammary glands	Mice – 5 pairs; rats – 6 pairs; extensive mammary tissue that extends to the neck and dorsum, only females have nipples	Guinea pigs – 1 pair; Chinchillas – 3 pairs	4 pairs with some variability	5 pairs
Scent glands	Rats and mice have preputial/clitoral glands adjacent to genital papilla; Syrian hamsters – paired flank glands; dwarf hamsters and gerbils-ventral midline gland	Guinea pigs have a "grease gland" dorsal to tail; Chinchillas have anal glands	3 pairs: chin glands, anal glans and inguinal glands; larger in males than females	Anal glands (removed if descended)
Male accessory sex glands	Seminal vesicles, coagulating glands, prostate gland, bulbourethral glands; hamsters also have ampullary glands	Seminal vesicles, prostate, coagulating glands, bulbourethral gland	Seminal vesicles, prostate gland, coagulating gland, proprostate gland, paraprostate gland, bulbourethral gland	Prostate (fusiform, 1.5 cm long)
Uterus	Long uterine horns, short body	Chinchillas have two cervices	Two cervices	Most pet ferrets are spayed
Vertebrae	7 cervical, 13 thoracic, 6 lumbar, 3–4 sacral and a variable number of caudal vertebrae	7 cervical, 13–14 thoracic, 6 lumbar, 203 sacral and 4–6 caudal vertebrae	7 cervical, 12–13 thoracic, 6–7 lumbar, 3 sacral, and a variable number of caudal vertebrae	7 cervical, 15 thoracic, 5 lumbar, 3 sacral and 18 caudal vertebrae
Brain	Lyssencephalic (no gyri and sulci)			Gyri and sulci

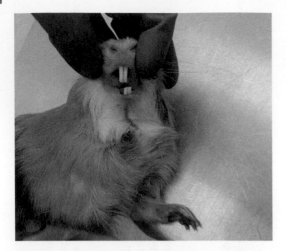

Figure 15.1 Malocclusion and overgrowth of teeth is a problem in rodents, so examination of the teeth is particularly important.

the ear canals and eyes provide five sections for histology that include most of the important structures of the head (Fig. 15.13). Eyes can also be removed and fixed separately.

Small organs (adrenal glands, lymph nodes) and soft organs (pancreas, thymus) should be put into cassettes for fixation. This will ensure that the small organs are not lost and that the soft organs fix flat, allowing more surface area for histology examination. As with cats and dogs, lymph nodes should always be labeled. Small hearts (mice, hamsters, gerbils) should be fixed whole, because the valves and chambers can be evaluated best on histologic sections, while larger hearts can be opened as described for the cat and dog. In small rodents, entire liver lobes, kidneys, spleens, and lungs can be fixed for histology.

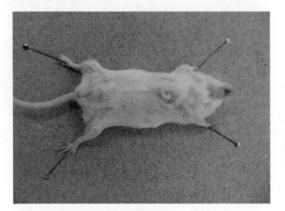

Figure 15.2 Pinning small mammals to a cork board can facilitate the necropsy procedure.

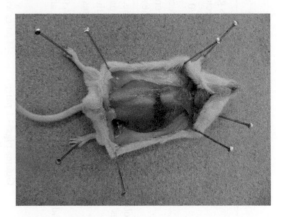

Figure 15.3 The skin is excised along the ventral midline and reflected.

(A)

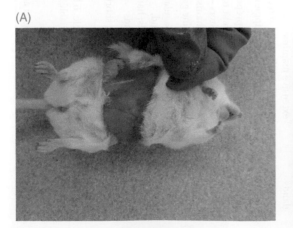

(B)

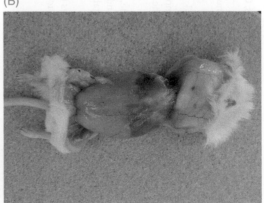

Figure 15.4 The skin can also be completely removed by making a small incision near the umbilicus, tearing the skin around the waist (Fig. 15.4A), degloving the skin cranially and caudally (Fig. 15.4B) and cutting the attachments around the ears, eyes, and anus.

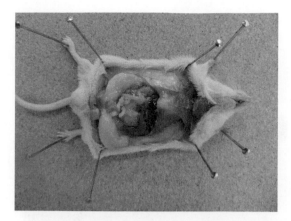

Figure 15.5 The abdominal cavity is opened by incising the body wall along the ventral midline and the costal margins.

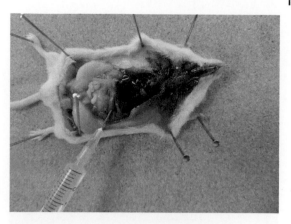

Figure 15.8 Formalin injection into the intestine facilitates fixation and inhibits putrefaction.

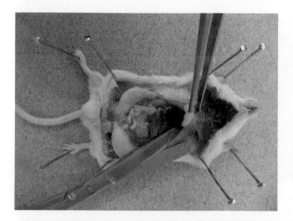

Figure 15.6 The thoracic cavity is opened by incising the ribs on both sides of the sternum.

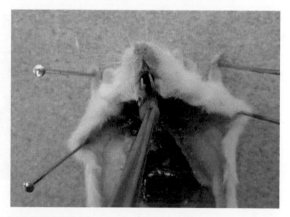

Figure 15.9 The mandibular symphysis is split with scissors and the tongue is extracted ventrally.

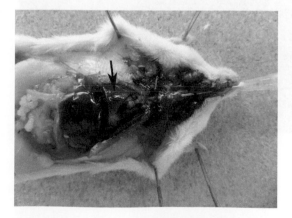

Figure 15.7 Insufflation of the lungs by injecting formalin into the trachea. Note the expanded lung (arrow).

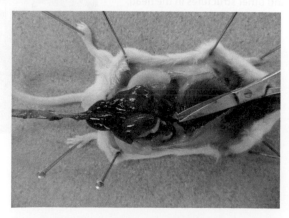

Figure 15.10 The periphery of the diaphragm is cut.

(A)

(B)

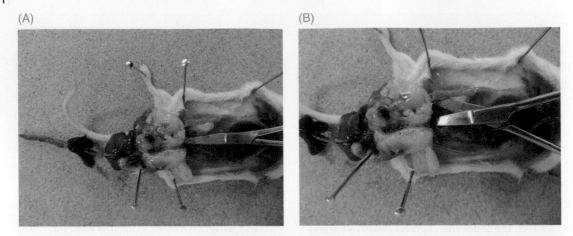

Figure 15.11 The pelvis is split by inserting closed scissors into the pelvic canal (A) and opening the blades (B).

Figure 15.12 All of the viscera are removed as a single unit (the "megapluck" or "superpluck").

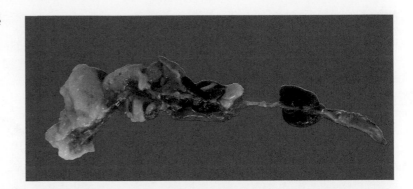

Figure 15.13 Sections of the decalcified head for histologic examination of the brain, eyes, ears, and other structures in the head.

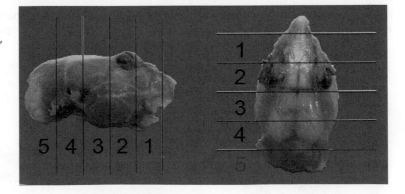

Bibliography

Brayton, C, Justice, M, Montgomery, CA. 2001. Evaluating mutant mice: anatomic pathology. *Vet Pathol.* 38:1–19.

Greenaway, JB, Partlow, GD, Gonsholt, NL, Fisher, KR. 2001. Anatomy of the lumbosacral spinal cord in rabbits. *J Am Anim Hosp Assoc* 37(1):27–34.

Holtz, W, Foote, RH. 1978. The anatomy of the reproductive system in male Dutch rabbits (*Oryctolagus cuniculus*) with special emphasis on the accessory sex glands. *J Morphol* 158(1):1–20.

Stan, F. 2015. Comparative anatomical study of lungs in domestic rabbits (*Oryctolagus cuniculus*) and guinea pigs (*Cavia porcellus*). *Bulletin UASVM Veterinary Medicine* 72(1):195–196.

16

Fetuses and Neonatal Animals

Necropsies of fetuses and neonatal animals are often unrewarding because these animals rarely have gross lesions. However, collection of samples for ancillary testing is critical for diagnosing or excluding infectious causes of abortion or neonatal death, and necropsies occasionally do reveal changes, such as congenital malformations, which provide important information for the owner or breeder.

16.1 Anatomy

16.1.1 Placenta

The cat and dog placenta is zonary and forms a band of tissue that encircles the fetus and attaches circumferentially to the wall of the uterus with the fetal membranes bulging out from both sides (Fig. 16.1). At the edges of the placental bands are pools of stagnant blood which grossly appear green and are referred to as the marginal hematoma. These bands are more pronounced in dogs than cats. Fetuses are usually equally distributed throughout the uterine horns; unequal distribution may indicate that a fetus was lost. The placenta is classified as endotheliochorial, meaning that the maternal endothelial cells are in contact with the chorionic epithelium. The weight of the canine placenta and newborn puppy vary considerably depending on breed. The feline placenta weighs 15–20 g without the umbilical cord or amnion and newborn kittens weigh 60–100 g.

16.1.2 Umbilical Cord

The canine umbilical cord is typically 7–8 cm long with few twists. It contains one vein and two arteries. The feline umbilical cord is 2–3 cm long and 0.3–0.5 cm in diameter with no twists. It contains two veins and two arteries, with no vitelline duct.

16.1.3 Fetal Circulation

An understanding of fetal circulation (Fig. 16.2) is important when necropsying a fetus or newborn animal. Oxygenated blood flows from the placenta to the fetus via the umbilical vein, which courses to the liver. Most of the blood bypasses the liver through the ductus venosus to the caudal vena cava. The blood flows to the right atrium, and much of the blood is shunted to the left atrium through the foramen ovale. Some blood does flow through the right atrioventricular valve to the right ventricle and into the pulmonary vein. Because the lungs are uninflated, the pulmonary vessels are collapsed and the majority of this blood is shunted through the ductus arteriosus to the aorta. Blood from the left side of the heart and the aorta flows to the rest of the body through the arterial system, capillaries and back to the heart through the veins. Some of the blood in the internal iliac arteries flows back to the placenta through the paired umbilical arteries. There is no direct mixing of fetal and maternal blood. Gas and nutrient exchange occurs between the maternal uterine vessels

Necropsy Guide for Dogs, Cats, and Small Mammals, First Edition. Edited by Sean P. McDonough and Teresa Southard.
© 2017 John Wiley & Sons, Inc. Published 2017 by John Wiley & Sons, Inc.
Companion Website: www.wiley.com/go/mcdonough/necropsy

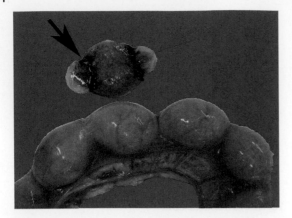

Figure 16.1 Canine uterus and placenta. The black arrow points to the marginal hematoma, at the edge of the zonary placenta. The red arrow points to the chorioallantois.

and the placental vessels much as it does in the lung, although much less efficiently. Gas exchange is driven by the high maternal blood flow to the placenta, the higher affinity for oxygen of fetal hemoglobin and the high hemoglobin concentration in the fetus.

16.2   Necropsy Technique

Before making the first incision, be sure to record the weight of the animal, the weight of the placenta, the length and number of twists in the umbilical cord or umbilical cord remnant (Fig. 16.3), the crown to rump length, and features of maturity such as fusion of the eyelids and ears, and presence of hair on the body (Table 16.1). In neonates, note the color and thickness of the umbilicus and check for urine staining indicating a patent urachus. If there is no fecal staining of the perineum, use a probe to check for patency.

Depending on the size of the animal, a fetus or neonate can be necropsied as described in Chapter 3, in left lateral recumbency, or as described in Chapter 15, in dorsal recumbency pinned to a corkboard.

Carefully examine the umbilical structures (Fig. 16.4) before removing the abdominal

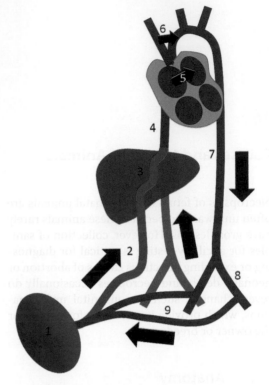

Figure 16.2 Schematic representation of fetal circulation. Oxygenated blood from the placenta (1) flows through the umbilical vein (2), and bypasses the liver through the ductus venosus (3), before mixing with unoxygenated blood in the caudal vena cava (4). Most of the blood entering the heart bypasses the lungs through the foramen ovale (5), between the right and left atria, or the ductus arteriosus (6), between the pulmonary artery and aorta). Blood flows through the aorta (7) to the iliac arteries (8). The umbilical arteries (9) arise from the internal iliac arteries and carry blood to the placenta.

viscera and cut around the umbilicus, leaving the umbilical arteries and urachus/urachal remnant attached. The bladder, urogenital tract, and umbilical arteries can be removed as a unit, opened and fixed.

Fetal ribs and skulls are often soft enough to cut with scissors. The skull bones may not be completely fused and may be somewhat distorted from the process of fetal expulsion. The young brain is poorly myelinated and very soft. It may even extrude from the foramen magnum as you attempt to cut the skull. If removing the

Figure 16.3 Feline fetus. Measurement of the crown to rump length and the length of the umbilical cord is recommended for all fetuses.

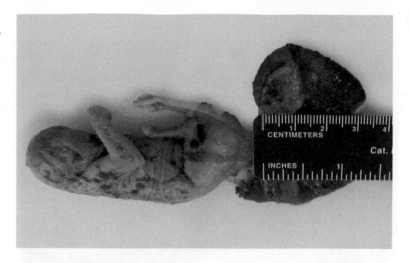

Table 16.1 Determining gestational age based on morphologic features.

Gestational Age (Days)	Crown to Rump Length (mm)	Fetal Characteristics
Feline		
20	10	Forelimb bud and otic vesicle present
24–26	18–20	Head touches heart bulge, olfactory pits form
27	25	Forelimb digits separate distally, pinnae triangular, eyelids forming
30	35	Tongue visible, digits widely spread, pinnae almost cover external meatuses
37	60	Claws forming, eyelids almost closed, pinnae cover external meatuses
43	80	Tactile hairs present on face
46	95	
50	110	Fine hairs cover body, claws hard and white, skin pigmented
55	125	
60	143	
60–63	143–150	Gestation complete
Canine		
30	20	Eyelids forming, grooves between digits, pinna partly cover external meatus, intestines herniate into umbilical cord
35	35	Eyelids partly cover eyes, pinnae cover external meatus, digits separated distally, external genitalia differentiated
38	55	Tactile hairs appear on upper lip and above eyes
40	60	Eyelids fused, intestines return to abdomen, claws formed
45	80	Body hair forming, color markings appear, digits separated
50	118	
53	140	Hair coat complete, digital pads present
57	160	
57–63	160–185	Gestation complete

From *Kirkbride's Diagnosis of Abortion and Neonatal Loss in Animals*, Fourth Edition. Published Online: December 22, 2011.

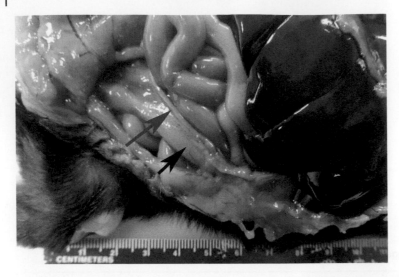

Figure 16.4 Newborn puppy. Examine the external and internal umbilical structures in all fetuses and neonates. The red arrow points to one of the umbilical arteries and the black arrow shows where the bladder blends with the urachal remnant.

brain is difficult, open up the calvarium, remove one eye and a portion of brain to save for possible ancillary testing, and fix the entire head.

The lungs of a fetus or stillborn animal are not aerated, are diffusely purple-red (plum colored) and sections will sink in formalin.

Always collect samples for ancillary testing and histopathology. The specific samples for abortion/neonatal death ancillary testing are covered in Chapter 19. The placenta is the most important diagnostic sample, and in the face of budgetary constraints, is the one sample to send for ancillary testing.

16.3   Common Artifacts and Postmortem Changes

Significant postmortem degradation is a common finding in fetuses (Fig. 16.5). The changes include discoloration of the skin and viscera, accumulation of clear and dark red fluid in the subcutis and body cavities, and sometimes

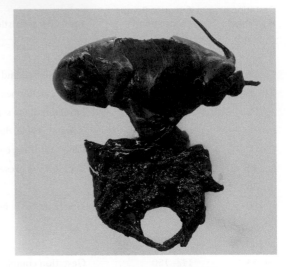

Figure 16.5 A severely autolyzed canine fetus. Although necropsy may be unrewarding, histopathology and ancillary testing may provide information about the cause of fetal demise.

emphysematous change. Alternatively, the fetuses can be shrunken, dark, and dry (mummified).

Part IV

Additional Testing

17

Cytology

Cytology refers to microscopic examination of fresh tissue preparations. Assuming a light microscope is available, cytology is a quick, inexpensive, and informative adjunct to the necropsy procedure. While most clinicians have some experience with cytology and are comfortable making basic diagnoses, unstained cytology slides can also be submitted to a board certified clinical pathologist who has extensive experience and knowledge in this area.

17.1 Types of Cytology Preparations

Traditional cytology preparations, such as blood smears, aspirates of masses, and fluid evaluation, can all be performed on postmortem samples. However, the workhorse of postmortem cytology is the touch imprint. While touch imprints of lesions are not a substitute for histology, these preparations allow for rapid evaluation of cellular morphology and often are helpful in identifying infectious agents and distinguishing between inflammatory and neoplastic conditions. Neoplastic cells can often be further classified as round, epithelial, or mesenchymal. The number of cells that adhere to the slide on a touch imprint depends on the tissue and the disease process. In a fresh cadaver, round cell tumors and inflammatory cells readily exfoliate, while touch imprints of sarcomas

and fibrotic tissue are usually paucicellular. The degree of exfoliation alone may be a clue to the nature of the disease process; however, in a postmortem sample, autolysis can also affect the propensity of cells to exfoliate.

17.2 Making a Touch Imprint

The first rule of making a touch imprint is use a clean blade to make a fresh cut into the area of interest. If a blade has previously been used to cut other tissues, cells and debris on the blade of the knife or scalpel will contaminate the imprint. Cut a small block (0.5–1 cm) out of the tissue of interest, cutting the surface to be used for the imprint first. Hold the tissue block with forceps and blot the surface with a clean paper towel (Fig. 17.1A). Touch the tissue gently to the slide multiple times, moving to a clean area of the slide for each imprint (Fig. 17.1B).

17.3 Making a Bone Marrow Smear

When collecting bone marrow for histology, it is easy to also make a smear of the marrow. Hematogenous cells undergo rapid autolysis, so the smear should be made as soon as possible. A moistened, clean, natural-bristle paint brush can be used to make a bone marrow

Necropsy Guide for Dogs, Cats, and Small Mammals, First Edition. Edited by Sean P. McDonough and Teresa Southard.
© 2017 John Wiley & Sons, Inc. Published 2017 by John Wiley & Sons, Inc.
Companion Website: www.wiley.com/go/mcdonough/necropsy

(A)

(B)

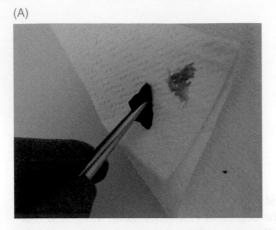 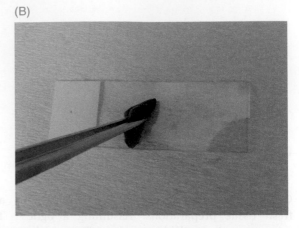

Figure 17.1 Making a touch imprint slide. Use a clean blade to cut a small piece of the tissue of interest. Blot the cut surface of the tissue several times on a clean paper towel (A). Lightly touch the cut surface of the tissue to a clean slide (B) and repeat on another area of the slide. Allow the slide to air-dry briefly prior to staining.

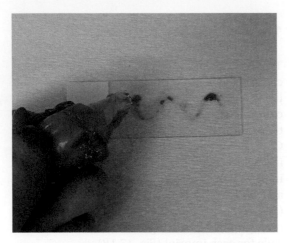

Figure 17.2 Making a bone marrow smear. Use the distal part of the femur, which has been opened to obtain a bone marrow sample for histology. Chip the cortex away from the cut end with bone cutting forceps and use the femur like a pencil to make a bone marrow smear.

smear. Alternatively, the distal femur, which has been opened to obtain the histology sample of bone marrow, can be removed and the cortex chipped away with bone forceps until the marrow is exposed. The femur can then be used like a pencil to make a serpiginous smear on a glass slide (Fig. 17.2). Forceps can also be used to hold a piece of bone marrow to make a smear.

17.4 Other Preparations

An unstained wet mount of feces can be examined for parasites and ova. Postmortem blood smears are not routinely done on small mammals, but are commonly used in species such as birds where hemoparasites are more common. Urine, CSF, synovial fluid, or effusion fluid can also be examined microscopically, although centrifugation is typically necessary to concentrate the cells, especially in CSF. If the smears cannot be made right away, the fluids should be stored in an EDTA tube.

17.5 Staining

The quickest and most practical stain for smears and touch imprints is Diff-Quik, which is a name brand of a modified Giemsa stain. This technique involves air drying the slide, then dipping it in three solutions: a fixative, the red Diff-Quik stain 1, and the purple Diff-Quik stain 2, followed by a quick rinse with tap water. The exact number and timing of dipping the slides varies slightly. The instructions on the kit say 30 s in each solution, but 10 quick dips in each also works. The staining characteristics of cells with Diff-Quik are shown in Table 17.1.

Table 17.1 Diff Quik staining properties of cells.

	Cytoplasm	Nucleus	Granules
Erythrocyte	Variable: pink, yellow-red or blue to purple		
Platelet	Obscured by granules		Violet or purple granules
Neutrophils	Pale pink	Dark blue to violet	Usually not apparent unless there is toxic change
Eosinophils	Blue	Blue	Pink
Mast cells	Light blue	Purple	Purple
Lymphocytes	Dark blue, light blue or clear	Violet	
Bacteria	Deep blue		
Other cells	Varying shades of blue	Blue to violet	

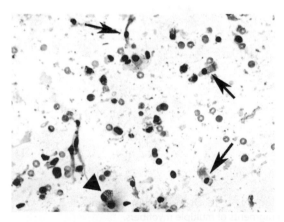

Figure 17.3 Touch imprint of the lung. Arrows point to ciliated respiratory epithelial cells. The arrow head points to an alveolar macrophage. Diff-Quik staining.

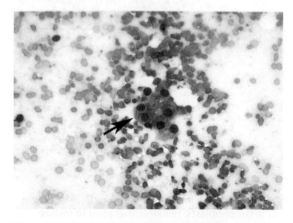

Figure 17.4 Touch imprint of liver. The arrow points to an aggregate of hepatocytes, surrounded by numerous erythrocytes.

Special stains, such as Gram, Ziehl–Nielsen, and Grocott's Methenamine silver (GMS) can also be done on cytology preparations.

17.6 Atlas of Normal Tissues

The images shown here (Figs. 17.3–17.15) are all taken from touch imprints of animals submitted for necropsy. These images may look somewhat different from the cytology pictures in textbooks. Those images are typically of aspirates from living animals which are fixed immediately. Autolysis affects the cellular structure as well as staining properties; however, even in these examples from animals with a postmortem interval of 6–24 h, cells can be identified and touch imprints can provide valuable diagnostic information.

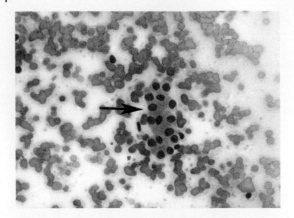

Figure 17.5 Touch imprint of kidney. The arrow points to a cluster of renal tubular epithelial cells, surrounded by many erythrocytes.

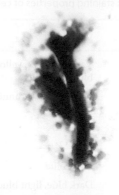

Figure 17.8 Touch imprint of heart. Two fragments of cardiomyocytes.

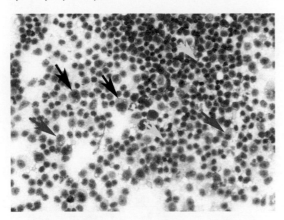

Figure 17.6 Touch imprint of lymph node. Black arrows pint to lymphoblasts. Yellow arrows point to mature lymphocytes. Red arrows point to plasma cells.

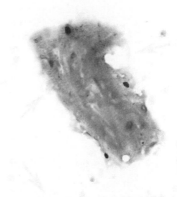

Figure 17.9 Touch imprint of skeletal muscle. Fragments of multiple myofibers.

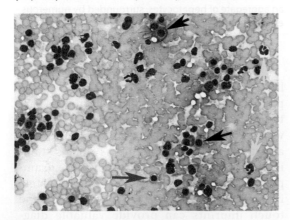

Figure 17.7 Touch imprint of spleen. Black arrows point to plasma cells. The red arrow points to a lymphocyte. Yellow arrows point to immature myeloid cells (extramedullary hematopoiesis).

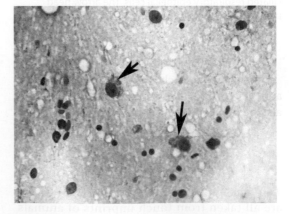

Figure 17.10 Touch imprint of cerebral cortex. Arrows point to neurons.

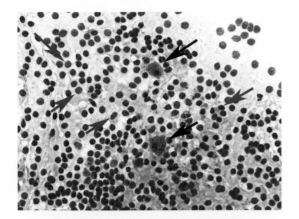

Figure 17.11 Touch imprint of cerebellum. Black arrows point to Purkinje cells. Red arrows point to granular cells.

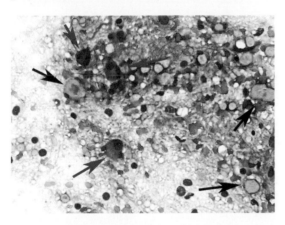

Figure 17.12 Touch imprint of spinal cord. Black arrows point to myelin. Red arrows point to surface epithelial cells.

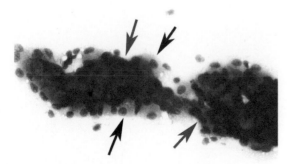

Figure 17.13 Touch imprint of stomach. Black arrows point to parietal cells. Red arrows point to chief cells.

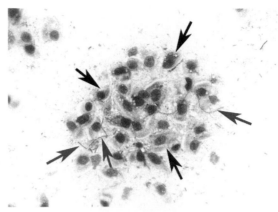

Figure 17.14 Touch imprint of small intestine. Black arrows point to mucosal epithelial cells (enterocytes). Red arrows point to bacteria (most likely postmortem overgrowth of *Clostridium* sp.).

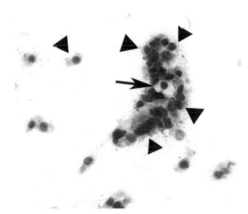

Figure 17.15 Touch imprint of colon. Arrow points to a goblet cell. Arrow heads point to mucosal epithelial cells (colonocytes).

18

Histopathology

Histopathology involves examination of stained sections of fixed tissues with the light microscope. Formalin-fixed samples submitted for histopathology are first trimmed into 2–3-mm-thick sections and placed in tissue cassettes. The tissues are then treated with a series of solutions containing increasing concentrations of ethanol to remove the water from the samples. A solvent (usually xylene) is used to displace the ethanol from the tissue and the tissue is infiltrated with paraffin wax and submerged in a mold filled with hot liquid wax, which is subsequently cooled down to form a solid block containing the tissue. The mold is removed and this block of wax and tissue is mounted to a microtome for sectioning. The microtome moves the block forward a set distance (the thickness of the desired section) and then down against a sharp blade to cut a thin (typically 3–5 um) section of the paraffin block and embedded tissue. Usually the block has to be sectioned several times or "faced" initially to create an even, flat tissue surface. The thin ribbon of wax and tissue cut by the microtome is placed in a water bath and scooped up on a glass slide. The wax is removed with xylene and the tissue is stained and covered with a coverslip. The routine stain used for histopathology is hematoxylin and eosin, but a whole array of other stains is available to highlight infectious organisms, extra and intracellular accumulations, fibrosis, certain cell types (such as mast cells), and basement membranes.

18.1 Necropsy Samples for Histopathology

The basic set of necropsy samples for histopathology is outlined in Appendix 3. Figure 18.1 shows the approximate size of samples that we routinely take for histopathology. The size of the samples needs to be large enough that the person trimming the tissues can recognize the sample for appropriate orientation, but small enough to fix completely.

18.2 Fixation

The quality of the histopathological diagnosis is only as good as the sample received. Tissues should be fixed as soon as possible. Sections should be no thicker than 0.5 cm and immersed in at least 10 times the volume of fixative. Proper tissue fixation is essential for obtaining diagnostically useful histologic tissue sections. Tissue fixation serves four functions:

1) Prevention of autolysis
   Cell death releases hydrolytic enzymes from lysosomes. The resulting autodigestive process greatly reduces cellular detail. Fixation acts by inactivating lysosomal enzymes and chemically altering the targets of lysosomal enzymes so that they are no longer susceptible to hydrolytic attack.

Necropsy Guide for Dogs, Cats, and Small Mammals, First Edition. Edited by Sean P. McDonough and Teresa Southard.

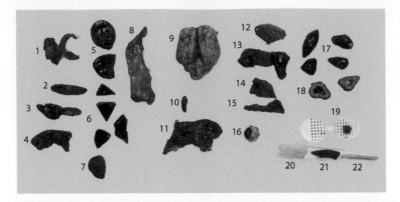

Figure 18.1 Necropsy samples for histopathology. 1. Esophagus and trachea; 2. Spleen; 3. Bone and bone marrow; 4. "T" section of heart (includes left ventricular free wall, septum and right ventricular free wall); 5. Right (transverse section) and left (longitudinal section) kidneys; 6. Liver, section from each lobe; 7. Tongue; 8. Urinary bladder (strip from apex to trigone); 9. Brain; 10. Thyroid gland; 11. Ilioceal junction and proximal colon; 12. Stomach; 13. Duodenum and pancreas; 14. Jejunum; 15. Distal colon; 16. Eye; 17. Lung, one section from each lobe; 18. Adrenal glands; 19. Pituitary gland; 20. Haired skin; 21. Skeletal muscle; 22. Sciatic nerve.

2) Insolubilization of tissue components

Proper fixation prevents tissue constituents from leaching out of the tissue during processing. No single fixative can insolubilize all tissue components, and lipids are especially difficult. Demonstration of lipids requires the use of either fresh or "wet" tissue (formalin fixed but not processed) and special stains (e.g., Oil Red O). Formal calcium is especially useful to preserve phospholipids. On the other hand, some insoluble components must be removed before certain tissues can be processed. Mineral salts of bone, which impart hardness to the skeleton, must be removed by decalcification before a section can be made.

3) Prevention of putrefaction

Devitalized tissue is an ideal environment for the growth of a wide variety of saprophytic bacteria and fungi. As they proliferate, these microorganisms produce substances that degrade tissue and reduce cytological detail.

4) Hardening of the tissue

Fixation stabilizes the cytoskeleton so that the tissue can resist deformation during trimming, dehydration, embedding, sectioning, and mounting.

There are five major groups of fixatives: (1) aldehydes, (2) oxidizing agents, (3) alcohol based fixatives (4) mercurials, and (5) picrates. The aldehydes (formaldehyde, glutaraldehyde) and oxidizing agents (osmium tetraoxide, potassium permanganate) fix tissue by cross-linking proteins. Formaldehyde reacts with primary amines to form Schiff bases and with amides to form hydroxymethyl compounds. The hydroxymethyl groups then condense with another amide moiety to form methyl diamides. Alcoholic hydroxyl forms acetals while sulfhydro groups form sulfhydral acetal analogues with formaldehyde. Based on the affinity to combine with formaldehyde, proteins are classified as having strong, moderate and low affinity. Tyrosine rings in proteins are the main determinant for the affinity of the protein to formaldehyde. Arginine, phenylalanine and tryptophan also contribute to protein affinity for formalin. Formaldehyde induced protein cross-links does not alter protein structure excessively and is good for immunohistochemistry, provided fixation is not prolonged. In contrast, glutaraldehyde deforms the alpha helix of proteins rendering them unsuitable for immunohistochemistry. However, glutaraldehyde fixation is very quick and 2% buffered glutaraldehyde is used primarily for electron microscopy.

Oxidizing agents also cause extensive denaturation of protein and thus are used very infrequently and only for specific purposes. Alcohol based fixatives (methyl alcohol, ethyl alcohol, acetic acid) are protein-denaturing agents (loss of quaternary, tertiary, and secondary structure) and are used primarily for cytology because they act quickly. Alcohols are seldom used for tissue fixation because they impart too much brittleness and hardness. The mercurial fixatives (B-5, Zenker's solution) form insoluble metallic precipitates (mercuric chloride) but the precise mechanism of fixation is unknown. Penetration of tissue by mercurials is poor, but fixation occurs quickly so very small samples can be fixed in as little as 30 min, although a minimum of two hours is generally recommended. Because they provide excellent nuclear detail, mercurial fixatives are used primarily for preservation of hematopoietic tissues (e.g., bone marrow and lymph node biopsies). Mercurial fixatives will corrode metal, including stainless steel and must be disposed of carefully because of their mercury content. B-5 Fixative zinc chloride is an alternative to B-5 with mercury but is very expensive. The primary picrate fixative is Bouin's solution. The mechanism of fixation by picrates is also unknown. Bouin's solution also produces excellent nuclear detail but does not induce as much tissue hardness as the mercurial fixatives. Bouin's solution is often used for biopsies of the reproductive tract and for fixing enucleated eyes. However, fixation must be limited to 24 h or the tissue will become too brittle to section. Regardless of the type, all fixatives should only be handled with gloved hands. Importantly, latex disposable gloves are permeable to most fixatives and the use of 4–8 mil nitrile gloves is recommended. Eye and face protection are essential when using mercurial or picrate type fixatives.

The most economical, reliable and readily available fixative is 10% neutral buffered formalin. Formaldehyde is a relatively volatile gas (boiling point, −21°C) but is very soluble in water and is obtained as a 37% solution known as formalin. For use as a fixative, formalin is diluted at a ratio of 1:9 to yield 10% formalin (3.7% formaldehyde). Formaldehyde is a polymer in concentrated aqueous solution but only the monomeric form is useful as a fixative. A 10% aqueous solution of formalin is very acidic (pH 2–4) and depolymerization is very slow. At neutral pH, depolymerization is rapid so formalin is best diluted in buffer to yield neutral buffered formalin. The acidity of formaldehyde is due to oxidation to formic acid. Methanol prevents formaldehyde oxidation so formalin should contain 1–2% methanol. In spite of the buffer, the solution will gradually acidify and 10% neutral buffered formalin should not be used if the pH drops below 6.5. Additionally, as formalin ages the concentration of methanol will increase. Methanol promotes denaturation of proteins, rather than cross linking, which can interfere with immunohistochemistry. Acid formaldehyde hematin consists of small, brown-black birefringent crystals formed by the action of an acidic formaldehyde solution on hemoglobin. Acid hematin occurs most commonly in the spleen, liver, lung, bone marrow, areas of hemorrhage, and blood vessels. Formation of formalin pigment cannot always be prevented by the use of buffered formalin, especially if fixation is prolonged. Ideally, 10% neutral buffered formalin should be used within 3 months of preparation.

Contrary to popular opinion, 10% neutral buffered formalin with methanol will freeze in cold weather and care should be taken when shipping formalin-fixed tissues during the winter. Wrapping the formalin jar in paper towels or newsprint and using an insulated shipping container are effective in reducing the chances of the specimen freezing during transport. In especially cold weather, it may be best to avoid shipping late in the week. Even insulated containers cannot prevent freezing if the box sits on an unheated loading dock for 2 or 3 days in sub-zero temperatures.

Formalin diffuses into tissue at a rate of about 1 mm per hour and fixative will completely penetrate a 0.5 cm thick tissue sample in 2–3 h. If the sections are too thick, the outer 1–2 mm will be properly fixed but the center of the tissue will be autolyzed. Importantly, penetration is not synonymous with fixation and complete fixation requires at least 24 h. If incompletely

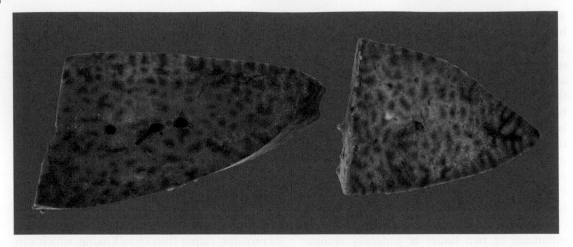

Figure 18.2 Samples of liver for histopathology. The sample on the left was too large, and the center remained unfixed (pink). The smaller sample on the right appears to be completely fixed; however, the color of the tissue changes before fixation is complete.

fixed tissue is processed, alcohol will fix the remaining unfixed tissue during processing by denaturing protein. While this will generate a histologic section of adequate quality, alcohol damages many protein epitopes, rendering the tissue unsuitable for immunohistochemistry. Note also that tissue exposed to formalin turns grey-brown well before fixation is complete and the color of the tissue should not be used to judge completeness of fixation (Fig. 18.2).

18.3 Practical Guidelines to Optimize Fixation

Autolysis begins as soon as the tissue is deprived of its blood supply (at the time of death or at biopsy). If immediate fixation is not possible, refrigerate the tissue. Do not freeze tissues since slow freezing produces damage due to the formation of ice crystals. Do not allow tissues to dry out since the artifacts produced are permanent and may obscure histopathological changes. Small sections of tissue are especially vulnerable to drying. Small samples are best placed in a tissue cassette rather than a red top tube or screw cap tissue bottle. Jostling during transport will often cause small tissue samples

to adhere to the lid, causing them to dry out. Specimens should be added to containers that already contain formalin to prevent adhesion of the tissue to the container. Swirling the specimen after a few minutes will help prevent adhesion and aid penetration. An adequate volume of fixative (at least 10:1) is essential since the effectiveness of the fixative will decline as its components are depleted due to fixation reactions. Always use fresh (within 3 months of preparation) 10% neutral buffered formalin with 1–2% methanol.

Clinicians often pressure the histology laboratory to speed up the process in order to get a quicker turnaround time. Increasing the temperature will increase the rate of penetration and the chemical reaction between the formaldehyde and tissue components. However, the increased temperature can increase the amount of autolysis in unfixed portions of the specimen. Microwave technology can be used for tissue fixation. In primary microwave fixation, fresh tissue in isotonic saline is irradiated. No chemical fixative is used at this stage. After microwaving, the tissues are immediately sliced to 2 mm and immersed in 70% ethanol. More commonly, microwave-assisted fixation is performed. The specimens are placed in buffered formalin before being microwaved. Microwave fixation must be carried out in a histology laboratory that can meticulously standardize every aspect of the procedure to ensure a suitable outcome.

On occasion, the veterinarian may wish to have a pathologist evaluate a large lesion or an entire organ, such as the heart or spleen. The best practice in these situations is to ship the entire fresh specimen chilled with gel packs by overnight courier. The organ should be placed in a plastic bag and then wrapped in paper towels or newspaper to prevent freezing. If this is not practical, digital photographs of the organ annotated with the location of representative sections is a viable alternative.

19

Infectious Disease Testing

The best sample for infectious disease testing is usually fresh tissue, body fluids, or swabs from areas of interest. However, many tests can be done on frozen tissue and some testing, such as immunohistochemistry and PCR, can be done on formalin-fixed tissue. Samples for these tests, unlike the samples for histopathology, do not need to be kept small, and often the ideal sample is a 3–4 cm cube of tissue. At the Animal Health Diagnostic Center, we have developed diagnostic plans for a variety of small animal conditions and those are summarized in Table 19.1. These can be modified based on the history and clinical presentation.

19.1 Test Types

A variety of different testing modalities are used for detecting infectious agents. Often there are multiple tests available for a single agent, which vary in terms of cost, turnaround time, sensitivity, specificity, and type of sample required. In general, it is always a good idea to check with the diagnostic laboratory where you will be submitting your samples prior to collection, to ensure you have the proper sample, and that it is stored and shipped appropriately. The following sections summarize the most common testing modalities for infectious agents.

19.2 Aerobic Culture

Aerobic culture involves swabbing the sample onto an appropriate bacterial growth medium, incubating the culture, and analyzing the resulting bacterial growth. Samples for aerobic culture should be collected as soon as possible after the body is opened and using clean (if not sterile) instruments. Aseptically collected swabs of tissues or fluids can be submitted in a specialized collection and transport system, which improves the survival of microorganisms if there is a delay in submission. Pieces of tissue can also be submitted in zipper lock bags or whirl packs. If tissue is submitted for culture, the surface(s) of the tissue are typically heat seared to kill off any surface contaminants. Most bacteria will grow on the standard bacterial culture media; however, some fastidious organisms require special media and, therefore, a special culture must be requested. These organisms include mycoplasma, brucella, yersinia and listeria. Salmonella cultures from enteric samples requires selective media to suppress overgrowth of other gastrointestinal coliforms. Laboratories that offer bacterial cultures often also provide additional testing for antibiotic sensitivity. For necropsy specimens, sensitivity testing is often not indicated unless other animals are affected or at risk.

Necropsy Guide for Dogs, Cats, and Small Mammals, First Edition. Edited by Sean P. McDonough and Teresa Southard.
© 2017 John Wiley & Sons, Inc. Published 2017 by John Wiley & Sons, Inc.
Companion Website: www.wiley.com/go/mcdonough/necropsy

Table 19.1 Infectious disease testing for dogs and cats.

Syndrome	Tissue	Canine Tests	Feline Tests
Diarrhea	Tied off loop of bowel (fresh or frozen)	*Campylobacter jejuni* culture Salmonella culture Clostridium difficile toxins (A/B) Parvovirus PCR, ELISA, FA Canine coronavirus PCR, FA Virus isolation Gram stain	*Campylobacter jejuni* culture Salmonella culture Feline coronavirus PCR, FA Feline parvovirus (panleukopenia) PCR, FA Virus isolation Gram stain
	Colon contents	Fecal qualitative Cryptosporidium ELISA Giardia ELISA Gram stain	Fecal qualitative Cryptosporidium ELISA Giardia ELISA Gram stain
Neurologic Signs	Consider referring case to a diagnostic lab or sending the entire head if animal is a rabies suspect or has bitten anyone		
	Meningeal or CSF swab	Aerobic culture Fungal culture	Aerobic culture Fungal culture
	CSF in red top tube	Aerobic culture Fungal culture Gram stain/fungal stain Virus isolation West Nile PCR Eastern equine encephalitis PCR	Aerobic culture Fungal culture Gram stain/fungal stain Virus isolation West Nile PCR
	Fresh brain tissue	Aerobic culture Fungal culture Fungal stain Virus isolation Canine distemper virus PCR	Aerobic culture Fungal culture Fungal stain Virus isolation
	Heart blood (do not freeze)	West Nile virus IgM capture ELISA	
	Complete transverse section of cerebellum and brainstem	Rabies FA	Rabies FA
	Fresh liver	Heavy metal screen	Heavy metal screen
Respiratory signs	Fresh lung	Aerobic culture Mycoplasma culture Fungal culture Fungal stain Virus isolation Canine distemper FA, PCR Canine parainfluenza FA, PCR Canine respiratory coronavirus PCR Influenza virus matrix PCR Canine herpesvirus FA, PCR Mycoplasma cynos PCR *Bordetella bronchiseptica* PCR Canine pneumovirus PCR	Aerobic culture Mycoplasma culture Fungal culture Fungal stain Virus isolation Chlamydophila FA, PCR Feline calicivirus FA, PCR Feline herpesvirus FA, PCR Influenza matrix PCR Feline parvovirus FA or PCR Feline pneumovirus PCR
	Feces	Qualitative fecal exam	Qualitative fecal exam

Table 19.1 (Continued)

Syndrome	Tissue	Canine Tests	Feline Tests
Abortion or neonatal death	Stomach contents	Aerobic bacterial culture (includes *Brucella canis*)	Aerobic culture
	Fresh lung	Aerobic bacterial culture (includes *Brucella canis*) Toxoplasma FA Virus isolation	Aerobic culture Feline herpesvirus FA, PCR Virus isolation
	Fresh Placenta	Aerobic bacterial culture (includes *Brucella canis*) Leptospirosis PCR, FA Virus Isolation	Aerobic culture Leptospirosis PCR, FA (rare in cats) Virus isolation
	Fresh Kidney	Leptospirosis PCR, FA Canine herpesvirus FA	Leptospirosis PCR, FA (rare in cats) Feline herpesvirus FA, PCR Virus isolation
	Fresh small intestine	Canine parvovirus FA, PCR	Feline parvovirus (panleukopenia) FA, PCR Virus isolation
	Fresh liver	Canine herpesvirus FA, PCR Virus isolation	Feline herpesvirus FA, PCR Virus isolation
	Fresh adrenal gland	Toxoplasma FA Virus isolation	Feline herpesvirus FA, PCR Virus isolation
	Fresh heart	Canine parvovirus FA, PCR Virus isolation	Virus isolation
	Thymus	Virus isolation	Virus isolation

19.3 Anaerobic Culture

Cultures for anaerobic organisms require special handling, since these organisms will not survive prolonged exposure to an oxygen rich environment. Specialized anaerobic culture collection systems are available to maintain the organisms during transport of swabs, small tissue samples or fluids/excreta. Anaerobic cultures can usually be performed from larger sections of tissue (3 cm or more) or ligated loops of bowel, if the tissue is kept refrigerated and delivered to the lab in less than 24 h. If delivery within 24 h is not possible, the sample should be promptly frozen and shipped frozen.

19.4 Fungal Culture

Fungal cultures can routinely be performed on the same sample types and sample handling conditions as for aerobic and anaerobic cultures. Bacterial transport media systems marketed for collection of clinical bacteria culture samples are also suitable for fungal culture. Fungal organisms grow slowly in culture; therefore, performing special stains for fungi on slide preparations of fresh or fixed tissue is indicated for a more expedient diagnosis.

19.5 Fluorescent Antibody Tests

Fluorescent antibody tests use an antibody tagged with a fluorescent marker to determine the presence of a particular antigen in a sample. These tests are often used to test for viral pathogens.

19.6 PCR

Polymerase chain reaction testing uses nucleic acid probes to detect and amplify specific segments of DNA. If the genetic material of interest is present, the PCR product will accumulate, allowing for detection.

19.7 ELISA

ELISA stands for enzyme-linked immunosorbent assay and uses enzymes linked to antibodies to detect a particular antigen.

19.8 Virus Isolation

Virus isolation involves exposing cultured cells to a sample of homogenized tissue in an attempt to infect the cells with a virus in the sample. The cultured cells are then evaluated for viral effects.

Virus isolation is similar to bacterial culture in that the laboratory generally is trying to culture and identify all significant, culturable viral pathogens consistent with the clinical history and gross findings of the case. However, not all viruses are routinely culturable from diagnostic submissions. Therefore, it is important to communicate with the diagnostic laboratory regarding viral agents in the differential diagnosis to determine if other testing modalities are necessary to substitute for or supplement virus isolation.

19.9 Qualitative Fecal

This is a microscopic examination of fecal material, often manipulated using osmotic gradients or centrifugation, in an attempt to identify parasites in the sample. Qualitative fecal examination differs from quantitative fecal examination in that parasite loads are not quantitated (counted).

19.10 Immunohistochemistry

Immunohistochemistry uses antibodies to identify antigens in histologic sections of tissue. Usually, immunohistochemistry is done in conjunction with routine histology examination of the tissue.

20

Toxicology Testing

Suspicion of malicious poisoning (usually by a neighbor) is a common reason for owners to request a necropsy for their pet. If unexpected death is defined as death occurring in an apparently healthy animal within a period of 12–24 h with no or minimal clinical signs, at least one study suggests that poisoning (accidental or purposeful) is the second leading cause of unexpected death in dogs. In cases where malicious poisoning is suspected, we recommend referring the case for a full gross and histopathologic examination by a board certified pathologist. If referral is not possible or if the case has no legal implications, this chapter covers the basics of collecting and submitting samples for toxicology testing.

Toxicology testing is relatively simple and reasonably priced if you know what you want to test for. However, tests to identify unknown toxins, such as mass spectrometry and liquid chromatography, tend to be much more expensive. Postmortem toxicology can determine whether a substance, such as a drug, is present in tissue, but often cannot determine how much of the drug was given, since the postmortem breakdown kinetics of most drugs are not known. Also, postmortem redistribution can greatly alter the concentration of a drug in a particular tissue. The best samples for toxicology are refrigerated or frozen (not fixed) pieces of tissue or fluids. We routinely collect 10 samples for possible toxicology testing (Fig. 20.1):

- Liver
- Kidney
- Spleen
- Lung
- Fat
- Brain
- Blood
- Urine
- Eye
- Stomach content

If a sample of feed or suspected bait is available, that should also be submitted. Ideally, 5–10 g of tissue, 2–4 ml of blood or 10–20 ml of other body fluids should be collected. These samples are stored in zipper lock bags or red-top tubes, and chilled or frozen until needed. Indications for common toxicology tests for small animals and appropriate samples are listed in Table 20.1.

Bibliography

Olsen, TF, Allen, AL. 2000. Causes of sudden and unexpected death in dogs: A 10-year retrospective study. *Can Vet J* 41:873–875.

Poppenga RH, Gwaltney-Brant S. 2011. *Small Animal Toxicology Essentials*. Hoboken, NJ: John Wiley & Sons, Inc.

Volmer PA, Meerdink, GL 2002. Diagnostic toxicology for the small animal practitioner. *Vet Clin NA, Small Animal* 32:357–365.

Necropsy Guide for Dogs, Cats, and Small Mammals, First Edition. Edited by Sean P. McDonough and Teresa Southard.
© 2017 John Wiley & Sons, Inc. Published 2017 by John Wiley & Sons, Inc.
Companion Website: www.wiley.com/go/mcdonough/necropsy

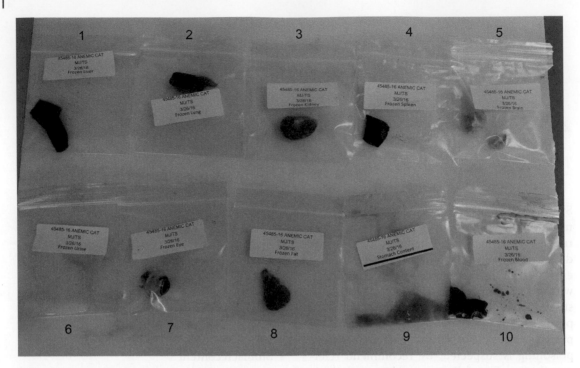

Figure 20.1 Recommended samples for toxicology testing. 1. Liver; 2. Lung; 3. Kidney; 4. Spleen; 5. Brain; 6. Urine; 7. Eye; 8. Fat; 9. Stomach contents; 10. Blood.

Table 20.1 Small animal toxicology indications and samples.

Agent	Clinical Signs	Gross Exam Findings	Sample
Ethylene glycol	Vomiting and anorexia, azotemia	Pale, swollen kidneys; Crystals on touch imprint	Liver, kidney, brain, blood
Anticoagulant rodenticide	Multifocal hemorrhages, anemia, melena, hematuria, hemoptysis, epistaxis	Multifocal hemorrhages	Liver, blood
Bromethalin rodenticide	Hyperexcitability, tremors, seizures, hyperthermia; Depression and weakness with lower doses	Usually none	Stomach contents, brain, liver, kidney, fat
Zinc	Anorexia, vomiting, diarrhea, lethargy, seizures	Icterus, hepatic necrosis, pancreatic hemorrhage	Liver, kidney
Mycotoxin	Varies depending on the specific mycotoxin; Aflatoxin causes inappetence, vomiting, depression, hemorrhage, icterus	Varies depending on the specific mycotoxin; Aflatoxin causes icterus, enlarged and firm liver, gall bladder edema	Liver, kidney
Copper	Acute: Abdominal pain, diarrhea, anorexia, hemolysis Chronic: Elevated liver enzymes, weight loss	Icterus, red urine, enlarged spleen, nodular liver	Liver, kidney
Lead	Anemia, blindness, seizures	Flattening or cerebral gyri, intestinal inflammation	Liver, kidney, blood
Arsenic	Diarrhea, vomiting, hemodynamic shock	Inflammation of intestinal mucosa	Stomach contents, liver, kidney, urine
Cyanide	Tachypnea, tachycardia, bitter almond breath, tremors	"Cherry red" blood and bitter almond odor, often no lesions	Liver, blood
Permethrin (cats)	History of tremors, seizures, depression, vomiting	No gross lesions	Urine, plasma, liver, fat, brain
Organophosphates and carbamates	History of salivation, lacrimation, urination, defecation, dyspnea, emesis (SLUDDE), bradycardia, tremors, coma, seizures	No gross lesions	Stomach contents, liver, kidney, brain, blood, eye
Organochlorine	Hypersensitivity, muscle fasciculation, tremors, seizures	No gross lesions	Stomach contents, liver, brain, fat
Alkaloids (Strychnine, caffeine, nicotine, theophylline, theobromine)	Tachycardia, hyperthermia, aggression, hypertension	No gross lesions	Liver, urine, kidney, stomach contents

21

Packaging and Shipping Samples

Formalin fixed samples must be shipped in a leak-proof primary container inside a leak-proof secondary container. The secondary container must be rigid and contain sufficient absorbent material (paper towels, cotton/cotton balls, cellulose wadding) capable of absorbing the entire liquid content. If shipping by air, the primary or secondary container must be rated for a 95 pKa pressure differential.

In contrast, when shipping clinical specimens that are known to contain or are reasonably expected to contain pathogens, the shipment must adhere to the regulations governing Biological Substances, Category B. All Category B infectious substances require triple packaging for shipment:

1) *Leak-proof Primary Container.* The specimen must be placed in a leak-proof primary container with a positive closure (e.g., screw-on cap). The volume of the primary container cannot exceed 500 ml (16.9 oz) for a liquid diagnostic specimen or hold more than 500 g (1.1 lbs) for a solid diagnostic specimen. When shipped by air, the primary or secondary container must be able to withstand a pressure differential of not less than 95 kPa (14 psi) in the range of −40–55 °C (−40–130 °F). For solid specimens, the primary receptacle must be sift-proof (i.e., the solid material cannot leak out of the packaging).

2) *Leak-proof Secondary Packaging.* To prevent contact between multiple primary containers, each must be individually placed inside a leak-proof secondary container. An example of the secondary container is a leak-proof biohazard bag. When shipping liquids, sufficient absorbent material capable of absorbing the entire contents of the primary container if it leaks must be included. An itemized list of contents must be placed between the secondary and outer containers and should be protected by storage in a leak-proof plastic bag (e.g., a Ziplock® bag). It is always advisable to check with the receiving laboratory for documentation requirements. Do not over pack the secondary container, as this may cause breakage of the primary containers. As a rule of thumb, a pencil should be able to fit between the primary containers after absorbent material is added.

3) *Outer Packaging.* The primary receptacle(s) and the secondary container(s) are placed inside a sturdy outer container that has a minimum of one rigid side 100 mm wide (4 inches, 100 mm × 100 mm). The outer container must consist of corrugated fiberboard, wood, metal, or rigid plastic and be appropriately sized for its contents. Place freezer blocks between the secondary container(s) when the specimens require refrigeration. For liquid specimens, the outer container must not contain more than a total of 4 l. For solid specimens, the outer container must not contain more than a total of 4 kg. Each complete package must be capable of withstanding a 1.2 m (4 foot) drop test outlined in IATA and DOT regulations.

Necropsy Guide for Dogs, Cats, and Small Mammals, First Edition. Edited by Sean P. McDonough and Teresa Southard.
© 2017 John Wiley & Sons, Inc. Published 2017 by John Wiley & Sons, Inc.
Companion Website: www.wiley.com/go/mcdonough/necropsy

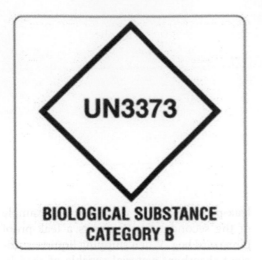

Figure 21.1 The outer container used to ship biological material must have a UN 3373 label.

The outer container must have a UN 3373 label with the words Biological Substance, Category B next to the diamond (Fig. 21.1). The outer container must also have the name, address and telephone number of the shipper, as well as the name, address and telephone number of the receiver/consignee. Category B shipments DO NOT require an Infectious Substance label, Shipper's Declaration for Dangerous Goods or emergency response information. (For details on shipping Category B infectious substances, visit: www.iata.org/NR/rdonlyres/ 9C7E382B-2536–47CE-84B4–9A883ECFA040/0/ Guidance_Doc62DGR_50.pdf.)

Although clinical specimens can be shipped with ice or dry ice, ice can leak in transit and dry ice is of concern to air transport carriers. The simplest way to keep clinical specimens cold is to use a sufficient number of frozen gel packs to keep the contents cool.

21.1 Packing Samples to Send to the Lab

When packing samples to send to the lab (Fig. 21.2):

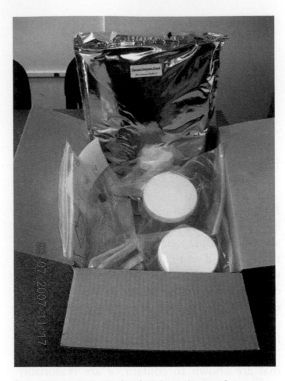

Figure 21.2 An example of triple packaging for shipment of Category B infectious substances. Individual specimens in leak proof containers are placed in leak-proof secondary containers. Before sealing the outer container, the samples are surrounded by absorbent material sufficient to absorb all the liquid contents should they leak.

- Include all items which must be chilled inside an insulated pouch or box
- Protect room temperature samples (Port-A-Cul®, Para-Pak®, Blood Culture) in a separate insulated container.
- Slides from impression smears should be placed inside an air tight plastic bag (e.g., a Ziplock® bag) to prevent exposure to formalin fumes and from becoming damp from condensation.

Bibliography

DOT 49 CFR Parts 171–180 (Online: www.ecfr. gov/cgi-bin/text-idx?tpl=/ecfrbrowse/Title49/ 49cfrv2_02.tpl, accessed August 17, 2016)

DOT Pipeline and Hazardous Materials Safety Administration: How to transport infectious substances (Online: www.phmsa.dot.gov/staticfiles/PHMSA/DownloadableFiles/Files/Transporting_Infectious_Substances_brochure.pdf, accessed August 17, 2016)

IATA Packing Instruction 650 – Biological Substances, Category B (Online: www.iata.org/NR/rdonlyres/9C7E382B-2536–47CE-84B4–9A883ECFA040/0/Guidance_Doc62DGR_50.pdf, accessed August 17, 2016)

Appendix 1

Normal Organ Weights (Percentage Body Weight)

Organ	Species	Age/Breed/Weight	Sex	Mean %BW	Reference
Adrenal glands	Cat	Newborn	Both	0.030%	Latimer, 1967
Adrenal glands	Cat	Adult	Male	0.014%	Northrup, 1960
Adrenal glands	Cat	Adult	Female	0.016%	Northrup, 1960
Adrenal glands	Dog	Adult (8–38 months, Beagle)	Male	0.006–0.013%	Latimer, 1967
Adrenal glands	Dog	Adult (8–38 months, Beagle)	Female	0.008–0.018%	Latimer, 1967
Adrenal glands	Dog	Newborn	Both	0.02%	Latimer, 1967
Brain	Cat	Newborn	Both	3.61%	Latimer, 1967
Brain	Cat	Adult	Both	0.80%	Bronson, 1979
Brain	Dog	Newborn	Both	2.74%	Latimer, 1967
Brain	Dog	Adult (8–38 months, Beagle)	Female	0.52–1.22%	Latimer, 1967
Brain	Dog	Adult (8–38 months, Beagle)	Male	0.54–1.05%	Latimer, 1967
Brain	Dog	Adult	Both	0.28%	Steward, 1975
Heart	Cat	Newborn	Both	0.77%	Latimer, 1967
Heart	Cat	Young (65 days)	Both	0.63%	Lee, 1975
Heart	Cat	Adult	Male	0.46%	Joseph, 1908
Heart	Cat	Adult	Female	0.46%	Joseph, 1908
Heart	Cat	Adult	Both	0.33%	Lee, 1975
Heart	Dog	Newborn (6–11 days)	Both	0.47%	Lee, 1975
Heart	Dog	Newborn	Both	0.76%	Latimer, 1967
Heart	Dog	Adult (9–20 months, Beagle)	Male	0.84%	Keenan, 2006
Heart	Dog	Adult (9–20 months, Beagle)	Female	0.85%	Keenan, 2006
Heart	Dog	Adult (mix breed, 0–10 kg)	Both	0.84%	Bienvenu, 1991
Heart	Dog	Adult (mix breed, >25.1 kg)	Both	0.72%	Bienvenu, 1991
Heart	Dog	Adult (mix breed, 10.1–25 kg)	Both	0.79%	Bienvenu, 1991
Heart	Dog	Adult	Male	0.74%	Joseph, 1908
Heart	Dog	Adult	Female	0.76%	Joseph, 1908

(*Continued*)

Necropsy Guide for Dogs, Cats, and Small Mammals, First Edition. Edited by Sean P. McDonough and Teresa Southard.
© 2017 John Wiley & Sons, Inc. Published 2017 by John Wiley & Sons, Inc.
Companion Website: www.wiley.com/go/mcdonough/necropsy

(Continued)

Organ	Species	Age/Breed/Weight	Sex	Mean %BW	Reference
Heart	Dog	Adult (8–38 months, Beagle)	Female	0.64%	Latimer, 1967
Heart	Dog	Adult (8–38 months, Beagle)	Male	0.65%	Latimer, 1967
Heart	Dog	Adult	Both	0.73%	Steward, 1975
Heart	Dog	Adult	Both	0.70%	Lee et al, 1975
Heart	Guinea Pig	Newborn (4 days)	Both	0.39%	Lee et al, 1975
Heart	Guinea pig	Adult	Male	0.42%	Joseph, 1908
Heart	Guinea Pig	Adult	Female	0.39%	Joseph, 1908
Heart	Rabbit	Newborn (1–3 days)	Both	0.49%	Lee, 1975
Heart	Rabbit	Adult	Male	0.27%	Joseph, 1908
Heart	Rabbit	Adult	Female	0.27%	Joseph, 1908
Heart	Rabbit	Adult	Both	0.20%	Lee et al, 1975
Heart	Rat	Newborn (12 hours)	Both	0.41%	Lee et al, 1975
Heart	Rat	Young (11–12 days)	Both	0.42%	Lee et al, 1975
Heart	Rat	Adult	Both	0.28%	Lee et al, 1975
Kidneys	Cat	Newborn	Both	1.06%	Latimer, 1967
Kidneys	Cat	Adult	Both	0.6–1%	Slatter, 2003
Kidneys	Dog	Newborn	Both	1.10%	Latimer, 1967
Kidneys	Dog	Adult	Both	0.60%	Slatter, 2003
Kidneys	Dog	Adult	Both	0.40%	Steward, 1975
Liver	Cat	Newborn	Both	4.07%	Nickel, 1979
Liver	Cat	Adult	Both	2.46%	Latimer, 1967
Liver	Dog	Newborn	Both	6.82%	Latimer, 1967
Liver	Dog	Young	Both	4.0–5.0%	Nickel, 1979
Liver	Dog	Adult (8–38 months, Beagle)	Female	2.5–3.9%	Latimer, 1967
Liver	Dog	Adult (8–38 months, Beagle)	Male	2.3–3.4%	Latimer, 1967
Lungs	Cat	Newborn	Both	2.53%	Latimer, 1967
Lungs	Cat	Adult	Not specified	0.62%	Watanabe, 1975
Lungs	Dog	Newborn	Both	2.97%	Latimer, 1967
Lungs	Dog	Adult (8–38 months, Beagle)	Male	0.62–0.85%	Latimer, 1967
Lungs	Dog	Adult (8–38 months, Beagle)	Female	0.61–0.85%	Latimer, 1967
Pancreas	Cat	Newborn	Both	0.24%	Latimer, 1967
Pancreas	Dog	Newborn	Both	0.23%	Latimer, 1967
Pancreas	Dog	Adult (8–38 months, Beagle)	Female	0.18–0.31%	Latimer, 1967
Pancreas	Dog	Adult (8–38 months, Beagle)	Male	0.15–0.43%	Latimer, 1967
Pancreas	Dog	Adult	Both	0.135–0.356%	Nickel, 1979
Spleen	Cat	Newborn	Both	0.17%	Latimer, 1967

(Continued)

Organ	Species	Age/Breed/Weight	Sex	Mean %BW	Reference
Spleen	Cat	Adult	Both	0.20%	Getty, 1975
Spleen	Dog	Newborn	Both	0.27%	Latimer, 1967
Spleen	Dog	Adult (8–38 months, Beagle)	Male	0.223–0.812%	Latimer, 1967
Spleen	Dog	Adult (8–38 months, Beagle)	Female	0.288–0.775%	Latimer, 1967
Thymus	Cat	Newborn	Both	0.30%	Latimer, 1967
Thymus	Dog	Newborn	Both	0.26%	Latimer, 1967

Bibliography

Bienvenu JG, Drolet R. 1991. A quantitative study of cardiac ventricular mass in dogs. *Can J Vet Res.* 55(4):305–309.

Getty R. 1975. *Sisson and Grossman's The Anatomy of the Domestic Animals*, 5th edn, Philadelphia, PA: Saunders.

Gronson RT. 1979. Brain weight-body weight scaling in breeds of dogs and cats. *Brain Behav. Evol.* 16:227–236.

Jackson B, Cappiello VP. 1964. Ranges of normal organ weights in dogs. *Toxicol Appl Pharma* 6:664–668.

Joseph, DR. 1908. The ratio between the heart-weight and body weight in various animals. *Jour Exper Med.*X:521–522.

Keenan CM, Vidal JD. 2006. Standard morphologic evaluation of the heart in the laboratory dog and monkey. *Toxicol Pathol.* 34(1):67–74.

Latimer HB. 1967. Variability in body and organ weights in the newborn dog and cat compared with that in the adult. *Anatom Rec.* 157(3):449–456,

Lee JC, Taylor FN, Downing SE. 1975. A comparison of ventricular weights and geometry in newborn, young, and adult mammals. *J Appl Physiol* 38(1):147–150.

Nickel R, Schummer A, Seiferle E. 1979. *The Viscera of Domestic Mammals*, 2nd edn. Berlin: Springer-Verlag.

Northrup DW, Van Liere EJ. 1960. Weight of adrenal glands of cats. *Proc Soc Exp Biol Med.*104:668–669.

Northup DW, Van Liere EJ, Stickney JC. 1991. The effect of age, sex and body size on the heart weight-body weight ratio in the dog. *Anatom Rec.* 128(3):411–417.

Slatter, DH. 2003. *Textbook of Small Animal Surgery, Volume 1*. Philadelphia, PA: Saunders. p. 1562.

Steward A, Allott PR, Mapleson WW. 1975 Organ weights in the dog. *Res Vet Sci.* 19(3):341–342.

Watanabe S, Frank R. 1975. Lung volumes, mechanics and single breath diffusing capacity in anesthesized cats. *J Appl Physiol* 38(6):1148–1152.

Appendix 2

North American Diagnostic Laboratories

This information was obtained from the American Association of Veterinary Laboratory Diagnosticians website (www.aavld.org/) and is current at the time of writing. Note that not all state diagnostic laboratories accept diagnostic samples from dogs and cats.

State	Address	Phone/Fax	Website
Alabama	Thompson-Bishop Sparks State Diagnostic Laboratory 890 Simms Road PO Box 2209 Auburn, AL 36832	Phone: 334–844–7207 Fax: 334–844–7206	http://labs.alabama.gov
Arizona	Arizona Veterinary Diagnostic Laboratory 2831 N. Freeway Tucson, AZ 85705	Phone: 520–621–2356 Fax: 520–626–8696	www.cals.arizona.edu/vdl
California	CA Animal Health & Food Safety Lab System UC Davis Shipping Address: 620 W. Health Science Dr. Davis, CA 95616 Mailing Address: PO Box 1770 Davis, CA 95617–1770	Phone: 530–752–8709 Fax: 530–752–5680	http://cahfs.ucdavis.edu
Colorado	Veterinary Diagnostic Laboratory Colorado State University Shipping Address: 300 West Drake Road Fort Collins, CO 80523 Mailing Address: 200 West Lake Street 1644 Campus Delivery Fort Collins, CO 80523–1644	Phone: 970–297–1281 Fax: 970–297–0320	www.dlab.colostate.edu

(*Continued*)

Necropsy Guide for Dogs, Cats, and Small Mammals, First Edition. Edited by Sean P. McDonough and Teresa Southard.
© 2017 John Wiley & Sons, Inc. Published 2017 by John Wiley & Sons, Inc.
Companion Website: www.wiley.com/go/mcdonough/necropsy

(Continued)

State	Address	Phone/Fax	Website
Connecticut	Connecticut Veterinary Medical Diagnostic Laboratory University of Connecticut Department of Pathobiology & Veterinary Science Shipping Address: 61 N. Eagleville Road, Unit-3089 Storrs, CT 06269–3089 Mailing Address: 61 N. Eagleville Road, Unit-3089 Storrs, CT 06269–3089	Phone: 860–486–3738 Fax: 860–486–2794	www.patho.uconn.edu
Florida	Florida Dept. of Agriculture & Consumer Services Shipping Address: 2700 N. John Young Parkway Kissimmee, FL 34741 Mailing Address: PO Box 458006 Kissimmee, FL 34745	Phone: 321–697–1400 Fax: 321–697–1467 Email:	http://doacs.state.fl.us
Georgia	Athens Veterinary Diagnostic Laboratory University of Georgia College of Veterinary Medicine 501 W. Brooks Dr. Athens, GA 30602–7383	Phone: 706–542–5568 Fax: 706–542–5977	www.vet.uga.edu/dlab
Georgia	Tifton Veterinary Diagnostic and Investigation Laboratory University of Georgia Shipping Address: 43 Brighton Road Tifton, GA 31793 Mailing Address: PO Box 1389 Tifton, GA 31793	Phone: 229–386–3340 Fax: 229–386–7128	www.vet.uga.edu/dlab
Illinois	Animal Disease Laboratory, Illinois Department of Agriculture Mailing Address: 2100 S. Lake Storey Road Galesburg, IL 61401	Phone: 309–344–2451 Fax: 309–344–7358	www.agr.state.il.us
Illinois	Veterinary Diagnostic Laboratory University of Illinois Shipping Address: 2001 South Lincoln Avenue, Rm 1224 Urbana, IL 61802 Mailing Address: PO Box U Urbana, IL 61802	Phone: 217–333–1620 Fax: 217–244–2439	www.cvm.uiuc.edu/vdl
Indiana	Animal Disease Diagnostic Laboratory Purdue University 406 South University St. West Lafayette, IN 47907	Phone: 765–494–7440 Fax: 765–494–9181	www.addl.purdue.edu
Iowa	Veterinary Diagnostic Laboratory, College of Veterinary Medicine Iowa State University Vet Diagnostic Laboratory 1600 S. 16th Street Ames, IA 50011	Phone: 515–294–1950 Fax: 515–294–3564	www.vdpam.iastate.edu

(Continued)

State	Address	Phone/Fax	Website
Kansas	Kansas State Veterinary Diagnostic Laboratory Kansas State University 1800 Denison Ave., Moiser Hall Manhattan, KS 66506	Phone: 785–532–5650 Fax: 785–532–4481	www.ksvdl.org
Kentucky	Breathitt Veterinary Center Murray State University Shipping Address: 715 North Drive Hopkinsville, KY 42240 Mailing Address: PO Box 2000 Hopkinsville, KY 42241–2000	Phone: 270–886–3959 Fax: 270–886–4295	https://breathitt. murraystate.edu/
Kentucky	Veterinary Diagnostic Laboratory- Lexington Shipping Address: 1490 Bull Lea Rd. Lexington, KY 40511 Mailing Address: PO Box 14125 Lexington, KY 40512	Phone: 859–257–8283 Fax: 859–255–1624	www.vdl.uky.edu/
Louisiana	LA Animal Disease Diagnostic Laboratory Shipping Address: 1909 Skip Bertman Dr. Rm. 1519 Baton Rouge, LA 70803 Mailing Address: PO Box 25070 Baton Rouge, LA 70894	Phone: 225–578–9777 Fax: 225–578–9784	http://laddl.lsu.edu
Michigan	Diagnostic Center for Population and Animal Health Michigan State University Shipping Address: 4125 Beaumont Road, Room 122 Lansing, MI 48910–8104 Mailing Address: PO Box 30076 Lansing, MI 48909–7576	Phone: 517–353–0635 Fax: 517–353–5096	www.animalhealth. msu.edu
Minnesota	Veterinary Diagnostic Laboratory University of Minnesota 1333 Gortner Avenue St. Paul, MN 55108–1098	Phone: 612–625–8787 Fax: 612–624–8707	www.vdl.umn.edu
Mississippi	Mississippi Veterinary Research and Diagnostic Laboratory System Mississippi State University Shipping Address: 3137 Highway 468 West Pearl, MS 39208 Mailing Address: P.O. Box 97813 Pearl, MS 39288	Phone: 601–420–4700 Fax: 601–420–4719	www.cvm.msstate. edu
Mississippi	The College of Veterinary Medicine Diagnostic Laboratory Services CVM-DLS (full service, all species) Veterinary Specialty Center 1207 Highway 182 W, Suite D Starkville, MS 39759	Phone: 662–325–7339 Fax: 662–325–3436	

(Continued)

(Continued)

State	Address	Phone/Fax	Website
Missouri	Veterinary Medical Diagnostic Lab University of Missouri Shipping Address: 1600 East Rollins Road Columbia, MO 65211 Mailing Address: PO Box 6023 Columbia, MO 65205	Phone: 573–882–6811 Fax: 573–882–1411	www.cvm.missouri. edu/vmdl
Montana	Montana Department of Livestock Montana Veterinary Diagnostic Laboratory Shipping Address: South 19th and Lincoln Bozeman, MT 59718 Mailing Address: PO Box 997 Bozeman, MT 59771	Phone: 406–994–4885 Fax: 406–994–6344	www. discoveringmontana. com/ liv/lab/index. asp
Nebraska	Veterinary Diagnostic Center PO Box 82646 Shipping Address: Fair Street, E. Campus Loop Lincoln, NE 68501–2646 Mailing Address: PO Box 830907 Lincoln, NE 68583–0907	Phone: 402–472–1434 Fax: 402–472–3094	http://vbms.unl.edu/ nvdls.shtml
New York	Animal Health Diagnostic Center College of Veterinary Medicine Cornell University Shipping Address: 240 Farrier Road Ithaca, NY 14853 Mailing Address: PO Box 5786 Ithaca, NY 14852		http://ahdc.vet. cornell.edu
North Carolina	North Carolina Department of Agriculture & Consumer Services Rollins Laboratory Shipping Address: 2101 Blue Ridge Road Raleigh, NC 27607 Mailing Address: 1031 Mail Service Center Raleigh, NC 27699–1031	Phone: 919–733–3986 Fax: 919–733–0454	www.ncagr.gov/vet/ ncvdl
North Dakota	Veterinary Diagnostic Laboratory North Dakota State University Shipping Address: Veterinary Diagnostic Lab Van Es Hall 1523 Centennial Blvd. Fargo, ND 58105 Mailing Address: NDSU Dept 7691 P O Box 6050 Fargo, ND 58108–6050	Phone: 701–231–8307 Fax: 701–231–7514	www.vdl.ndsu.edu
Ohio	Animal Disease Diagnostic Lab 8995 E. Main Street, Building 6 Reynoldsburg, OH 43068	Phone: 614–728–6220 Fax: 614–728–6310	www. ohioagriculture.gov/ addl

(Continued)

State	Address	Phone/Fax	Website
Oklahoma	Oklahoma Animal Disease Diagnostic Laboratory Oklahoma State University Shipping Address: Center for Veterinary Health Sciences Farm and Ridge Road Stillwater, OK 74078 Mailing Address: PO Box 7001 Stillwater, OK 74076–7001	Phone: 405–744–6623 Fax: 405–744–8612	www.cvm.okstate. edu
Oregon	Veterinary Diagnostic Laboratory Oregon State University Magruder Hall, Room 134 Shipping Address: 30th and Washington Way Corvallis, OR 97331 Mailing Address: 134 Magruder Hall, Corvallis OR 97331	Phone: 541–737–3261 Fax: 541–737–6817	http://vetmed. oregonstate.edu/ diagnostic
Pennsylvania	Department of Agriculture Pennsylvania Veterinary Laboratory 2305 N. Cameron Street Harrisburg, PA 17110–9408	Phone: 814–863–0837 Fax: 814–865–3907	www.padls.org
South Dakota	Animal Disease Research and Diagnostic Laboratory South Dakota State University Shipping Address: Animal Disease Research Building, North Campus Drive Brookings, SD 57007–1396 Mailing Address: Box 2175, North Campus Drive Brookings, SD 57007–1396	Phone: 605–688–5171 Fax: 605–688–6003	http://vetsci.sdstate. edu
Tennessee	CE Kord Animal Health Diagnostic Laboratory Ellington Agriculture Center Shipping address: 440 Hogan Rd. Porter Building Nashville, TN 37220 Mailing address: PO Box 40627 Nashville, TN 37204	Phone: 847–714–2753 Fax: 615–837–5250	www.state.tn.us/ agriculture/regulate/ labs/kordlab.html
Texas	Texas A&M Veterinary Medical Diagnostic Laboratory (TVMDL) TVMDL-College Station Shipping Address: 1 Sippel Road College Station, Texas 77843 Mailing Address: P.O. Drawer 3040 College Station, TX 77841–3040	Phone: 979–845–3414 Fax: 979–845–1794	http://tvmdl.tamu. edu
Utah	Utah Veterinary Diagnostic Laboratory Utah State University 950 East 1400 North Logan, UT 84341	Phone: 435–797–1885 Fax: 435–797–2805	www.usu.edu/uvdl

(Continued)

(Continued)

State	Address	Phone/Fax	Website
Washington	Washington Animal Disease Diagnostic Laboratory Washington State University Shipping Address: Hall Room 155 N Pullman, WA 99164–7034 Mailing Address: PO Box 647034 Pullman, WA 99164–7034	Phone: 509–335–6047 Fax: 509–335–7424	www.vetmed.wsu.edu/depts_waddl
Wisconsin	Wisconsin Veterinary Diagnostic Laboratory University of Wisconsin 445 Easterday Lane Madison, WI 53706	Phone: 608–262–5432 Fax: 847–574–8085	www.wvdl.wisc.edu
Wyoming	Wyoming State Veterinary Laboratory 1174 Snowy Range Road Laramie, WY 82070	Phone: (307) 766–9925 Fax: (307) 721–2051	
Canada	Animal Health Laboratory University of Guelph Shipping Address: 419 Gordon Street NW Corner Gordon/McGilvray Guelph, Ontario N1G 2 W1 Mailing Address: PO Box 3612 Guelph Ontario N1H 6R8, Canada	Phone: 519–824–4120 Fax: 519–827–0961	http://ahl.uoguelph.ca
Canada	The Animal Health Centre 1767 Angus Campbell Road Abbotsford, BC V3G 2 M3 Canada	Phone: 604–556–3003 Fax: 604–556–3010	www.agf.gov.bc.ca/ahc/
Canada	University of Montreal Diagnostic Services Faculte de medecine veterinaire Shipping Address: 3200 rue Sicotte Saint-Hyacinthe, Quebec Canada J2S 2 M2 Mailing Address: C. P. 5000 Saint-Hyacinthe Quebec. J2S 7C6, Canada	Phone: 450–773–8521 Fax: 450–778–8107	www.medvet.umontreal.ca/RCTLSA/program.html

Appendix 3

Tissue Collection Checklist

Standard Set of Tissues for Histopathology

- All lesions
- Peripheral nerve
- Skin
- Skeletal muscle
- Bone and bone marrow
- Any enlarged lymph node, labeled with location
- Tongue
- Trachea
- Esophagus
- Thyroid glands with parathyroids, in a cassette if small
- Thymus
- Lung, one section from each lobe
- Heart, either whole heart or sections from left ventricle, right ventricle, and septum
- Liver, one section from each lobe
- Gall bladder, if not included with liver section
- Spleen
- Adrenal glands, in a cassette if small
- Kidney, longitudinal section from left, transverse section from right
- Urinary bladder, longitudinal strip with apex and trigone
- Prostate gland (males)
- Gonads
- Uterus, entire or sections of body, and horn (females)
- Stomach, longitudinal strip that includes cardia, body, pylorus, or samples of each part
- Duodenum and pancreas

- Jejunum
- Ileocecocolic junction and lymph node
- Proximal colon
- Distal colon
- Brain, entire brain except for any sections collected for other tests
- Pituitary gland
- Eye

Additional Tissues for Histopathology, if History Warrants

- Larynx
- Pharyngeal tonsils
- Urethra
- Ureter
- Penis
- Vagina
- Aorta
- Pulmonary artery
- Additional peripheral nerves
- Additional sections of skeletal muscle
- Additional sections of bone
- Joint capsule
- Additional sections of skin
- Nasal cavity section
- Petrous temporal bone section
- Mammary gland
- Anal sac
- Diaphragm
- Salivary gland

Necropsy Guide for Dogs, Cats, and Small Mammals, First Edition. Edited by Sean P. McDonough and Teresa Southard.
© 2017 John Wiley & Sons, Inc. Published 2017 by John Wiley & Sons, Inc.
Companion Website: www.wiley.com/go/mcdonough/necropsy

- Tendon
- Ligament
- Spinal cord
- Ganglia
- Cranial nerves

Samples for Toxicology

- Blood
- Urine
- Stomach contents
- Lung
- Liver
- Kidney
- Spleen
- Brain
- Eye
- Adipose tissue

Samples for Infectious Disease Testing

Abscess

- Swab of contents

Respiratory Disease

- Fresh lung
- Feces
- Tracheobronchial lymph node

Diarrhea

- Tied off loop of bowel
- Colon contents

Abortion

- Stomach contents
- Fresh lung
- Fresh placenta
- Fresh kidney
- Fresh small intestine
- Fresh adrenal gland
- Fresh heart
- Fresh thymus

Neurologic Disease

- Meningeal or CSF swab
- CSF in red top tube
- Fresh brain
- Heart blood
- Fresh liver

Appendix 4

Describing Gross Lesions

A4.1 Color

Red – Hemorrhage, Congestion, Hemoglobin Staining (Imbibition)

White – Mineral, Fat, Fibrous Tissue, Absence of Blood Flow, Necrosis

Green – Bile Staining, Putrefaction, Eosinophilic Inflammation

Yellow – Bilirubin (Icterus), Hematoidin (Erythrocyte Breakdown), Carotenoids (High Vitamin A Diet)

Brown – Hemosiderin/Iron Deposition, Methemoglobin, Lipofuscin

A4.2 Consistency

Soft – Necrosis, adipose tissue, lung

Firm – Inflammation, fibrosis, cartilage

Hard – Mineralization, bone

A4.3 Demarcation

Well demarcated – vascular insult, benign tumor

Poorly demarcated – inflammation, malignant tumor

A4.4 Contour

Sessile – having a broad base

Pedunculated or polypoid – having a narrow base

A4.5 Shape

Round – benign tumor, vascular (some organs), cystic lesion

Rectangular or polygonal – vascular (some organs such as skin)

Irregular – malignant tumor, inflammatory process

A4.6 Distribution

Focal – primary tumor, traumatic injury, early stage of multifocal process

Multifocal – hematogenous spread of infectious agent or neoplasm

Multifocal to coalescing – Progression of multifocal lesion

Locally extensive – Vascular insult, progression of focal lesion

Diffuse – Metabolic, progression of multifocal or locally extensive lesion, vascular insult

Necropsy Guide for Dogs, Cats, and Small Mammals, First Edition. Edited by Sean P. McDonough and Teresa Southard.
© 2017 John Wiley & Sons, Inc. Published 2017 by John Wiley & Sons, Inc.
Companion Website: www.wiley.com/go/mcdonough/necropsy

A4.7 Fluid

Watery – serum
Viscous – contains mucous or fibrin
Turbid – contains fibrin, inflammatory or neo-
plastic cells
Opaque – contains cells or lipid droplets

A4.8 Shape

Circular	Ovoid	Pyramidal
Spherical	Cylindrical	Wedge shaped
Ellipsoid	Triangular	Conical
Rectangular	Linear	Reniform
Polygonal	Fusiform	Spatulate
Trapezoidal	Oblong	Polypoid
Multifaceted	Lancet-shaped	Stellate
Concave	Lenticular	
Convex	Cordate	

A4.9 Lesion borders

Sharp	Dentate	Circumscribed
Angulated	Sawtooth	Indistinct
Clefted	Serrate	Interdigitated
Semilunar	Lobed	Pedunculated
Curvilinear	Papillary	Sessile
Pinnate	Villous	Filamentous
Serpiginous	Infiltrating	Fimbriated

Bibliography

King JM, Roth-Johnson L, Dodd DC, Newson
ME. 2005. *The Necropsy Book*. Gurnee, IL;
CL Davis DVM Foundation Publishers.
Schmidt, WA. 2007. *Principles and Techniques
of Surgical Pathology*. Menlo Park, CA:
Addison-Wesley Publishing Company,
pp. 708–729.

Index

Necropsy Guide for Dogs, Cats, and Small Mammals, First Edition. Edited by Sean P. McDonough and Teresa Southard.
© 2017 John Wiley & Sons, Inc. Published 2017 by John Wiley & Sons, Inc.
Companion Website: www.wiley.com/go/mcdonough/necropsy

Printed and bound by CPI Group (UK) Ltd, Croydon, CR0 4YY

27/10/2024